UNDERSTANDING THE
EPIDEMIC

+ the (not so) elusive solutions

———————

Written by Cleaus Neverson-Browne

———

Contents

Preface

I believe that natural therapies and practices should and have the capability to be at the forefront of mainstream healthcare and because of this my contribution to making this happen is through empowering natural healthcare practitioners of all kinds, empowering the general public with the knowledge and tools they need to make this a living reality and anything else I can do to manifest this worthwhile goal into our world today. This book stems from that belief and vision.

So, why should you take the time to read this book?

Well, just like me, you have probably looked around and at some point asked yourself the question:

"Why is everyone getting so sick nowadays?"

That is a very valid question and one we aim to address through out this book. We are seeing an unprecedented rise in a wide range of diseases all happening at the same time. Why is this?

- In the western world, 1 in 3 people are expected to get cancer at some point in their lifetime

- Hundreds of thousands of people are affected every year by some form of autoimmune disease

- Hundreds of thousands of people are dying from diabetes related deaths each year

- Even more die from cardiovascular related diseases every year too

... And the list goes on and all of these numbers are predicted to rise as we move into the future.

Would you agree then that it is important for us to understand why this is happening and to see if there is anything we can do about it?

If you do agree with this, then this book will be more than beneficial to you.

In this book we address the rising epidemics of these diseases, their causes and what is happening within the human organism with regards to them.

We will then address the core essentials that the body needs in order for all of its systems to function at its full capacity. We will look at the nervous system and break this down so we can understand its underlying function and we will do the same with the immune system.

The premise here is that if we understand how the body functions from its deepest level, we can better understand what needs to be done to bring it back to full vitality and out of disease.

Once we have addressed these important issues, we then take you through the most prevalent diseases facing our societies today one by one and address their causes and walk through their solutions to begin the journey back to full vibrant health.

Now, even though this book mainly addresses the problems we are seeing in western societies, much of the issues we discuss here are actually slowly being adopted by the rest of the world and so this book is still very relevant to people all over the world that must be on the look out for such things.

I hope you will come with us on this journey of exploration as we start: *Understanding The Epidemic and the (not so) elusive solutions.*

Introduction

I wanted to start this book with just a bit of context as to where the idea to write this book in particular actually came from and what I hope to get across to you by the end of it. My hope in doing this is that it will invoke in you the same kind of questioning and inquisitive nature that has come to be part of my daily life coupled with the refusal to take things at face value.

I'll give you the short version of how it all came to be.

My personal journey of natural health began a few years ago in 2012. It was at this time that I started thinking more about what I was doing and the direction in which I wanted my life to go.

As you will probably remember, 2012 was the big hype about 'the end of the world' on 21st December of that year. So just out of interest and wanting to understand where all of this talk was coming from I started looking into the Mayan civilisation as this idea of something ending on this date came from a calendar that they had written a long time ago.

Now, to be honest, I didn't have a clue if this was real or if it was something made up. But I know one thing is for sure, as I was continually hearing about it, it actually made me question my mortality.

It made me wonder:

> 'What if the world actually does end? what actually happens next? What happens after

death? Even if this isn't the end of the world like they say, what happens if I was actually to drop dead tomorrow?'

These and a load of other similar questions started to come up in my mind.

I had thought of these types of questions before just messing around with friends or in passing, but never gave them any real thought. I just thought of it as:

'Oh, I'm young, that's not going to happen for a long time'

But then as this whole situation came along it made me think that it could be closer than I may have first thought.

This led me to want to learn more about life in general, our planet, death and other related subjects just because I really didn't pay much attention to it before. Yet these were very important topics for any person to consider.

This also then continued into me wanting to learn more about myself, what I wanted and had been doing up until this point, what made me happy and what, if the world didn't end, I could see myself happily doing for the rest of my life.

Looking back, I can't remember if it was a conscious choice or not, but it was around this time that I started really getting into spirituality and the concepts surrounding this. During this early exploration I came across the fascinating art of energy healing and some of the amazing results that people had seen after using this form of healing.

Many people in the west today, especially the medical establishments, would brush this aside as being rubbish, but in the east they have entire hospitals and thousands of centres dedicated to it with some really fascinating results.

I had heard about Reiki before but I didn't really understand what it was or how it worked and so became intrigued with it all. I set out to learn how to do energy healing myself to see if it really did work the way people had claimed. I found a course and began to study and learn one modality of energy healing called Pranic Healing.

I was so amazed and actually quite surprised that it really did work.

I started getting testimonials from people saying how in some cases they had stopped taking the strong pain killers they were on because of our time working together and, one that really stuck with me, that my little cousin who had Asthma since she was born and had to use an inhaler multiple times daily, now didn't have to use one at all, she could run and do P,E at school again and could run around on the playground with her friends without getting out of breath and wheezy.

This was after just two of our healing sessions… But I digress. This book is not actually about energy healing, so I will continue.

I carried on the practice and started helping a range of other people with their physical and psychological ills and continue to this day and have found this practice to be so rewarding.

But I wasn't quite finished there. Since this exploration started, I have been continually just learning and learning and wanting to grow and develop as much as I can. This became a snowball type effect of learning and enquiring into natural health concepts and practices that led me to a wide range of discoveries relating to health.

These discoveries included things like:

- Understanding the pharmaceutical industry. How it works, its history and its effect and place in our lives

- Understanding different approaches to healthcare - the good and the bad

- Understanding why certain things work while others don't with regards to healthcare

- Understanding some really important core factors that affect our health and wellbeing

- Understanding some fundamental facts about the body

- Understanding the use of food and diet in repairing the body and bringing it back to full health

- Understanding the workings of the inside of this universe of a body we inhabit and how things are interconnected and interdependent within it

- Understanding how to address certain problems with some simple and straight forward concepts

- Understanding why the world is seeing the amount of diseases we see today and what we can do about it

All of these things and more I have learned, researched and come to realise and this is what I aim to get across in this book for you.

This book is not about energy healing, but about:

- How this human body functions

- What this human body needs on a physical level

- What internally and externally can affect it

- Understanding how and why todays epidemic of diseases have come about and

- What we can do about it to reduce this impact

The idea behind listing the conditions and diseases out in A-Z format actually came about because I was going to use this as a reference guide for personal use.

A place where I could come back and refresh my memory with all the topics and interesting findings that I had been uncovering and learning.

As soon as I started writing though I quickly realised that this would not only benefit myself but could be used by healers, healthcare professionals and the general public the world over. So I decided to write this book as you see it today.

It is a culmination of a wide range of things I have been looking into and learning with regards to physical health for a while now and so I hope it brings you as much knowledge, understanding and help as it has brought me and those that I have worked with.

All of the concepts, techniques and recommendations in this book are not my personal opinion, but the known successful practices of naturopaths, alternative medicine practitioners and an increasing number of medical doctors around the globe today.

The conditions that are listed in this book are the most common physical conditions and diseases that we see in the world today, many of which have exploded in the number of cases diagnosed in the last 20 – 25years.

I am sure that you will know of someone in your life that has a problem with at least one of these conditions.

If not, you are in the minority group.

For each condition we will address what they are, how they come about in the first place and what we can do to work towards naturally reducing their impact, eradicating them out of our lives altogether and/or preventing ourselves from getting into these situations in the first place.

I thought I would keep the subjects of depression and anxiety and other related psychological disorders for separate book.

The aim of this book is to help us all understand how the body functions a little better. The thinking behind this is that if we understand how the body works under certain conditions and how it reacts to internal and external changes, we can better understand the causes and solutions to our dis-eases (a state in which the body is not at ease or in natural balance).

You will notice that as you read through the book, in a lot of the sections, I will be repeating key important points. This is not by accident. I do this for these three core reasons:

1. The body works and has worked in pretty much the same way for thousands of years. Yes, different diseases have come and gone and we may have developed new means to deal with them, but ultimately the biology of the body works in a certain way.

If you give the body the right internal and external environment and the right raw materials that it needs, it will generally do the rest for you by keeping everything balanced and healthy and it does a very good job of this too.

The body has an innate ability for self-preservation.

This is not to say that everyone is exactly the same

and needs exactly the same things in exactly the same quantities, but just to understand that there are certain things that every human body needs and this is what I have tried to present in this book.

2. By repeating points over and over, it will more likely stick with you, the reader. This is because repetition really is the father of learning, something that I'm sure you have all heard time and time again.

Repetition helps to solidify something into the subconscious mind a lot quicker where it will then be stored and more likely acted upon than otherwise.

3. Finally, I will assume that some of you will just jump to the condition you want to know about and may not read the entire book straight away and because of this I had to include all of the information that is relevant to that condition. This is so you will have all the info you need without having to read the entire book.

You will also notice that at times I will refer you to other sections of the book where we have gone into further detail about a given solution or explanation. This is just so the book is no longer than it needs to be.

I would also like to say that this book is not here to fight against the medical establishments of pharmaceutical companies and doctors. That is not the intention of this book.

I fully agree that in severe cases medical intervention is needed but I also believe that natural methods should always be sought after first in an attempt to assist the body to heal itself in a natural and holistic way.

Generally, when the body has a problem or disease, it is not the body turning on you or just malfunctioning, but its attempt to adjust to the new environment that has been established within it.

The body makes these changes, say for example in blood sugar and blood pressure, in order to keep everything functioning the way it needs to be and many times medications can suppress this natural response rather than fix the core of what caused these changes. This is another reason why I believe natural methods that treat the core cause should always be explored first and then in severe cases medical intervention should be considered.

I firmly believe, and it has been shown in various studies and cases, that most parts of the body can regenerate and heal when given the right environment internally and externally and when given the right nutrition and care.

I want to personally thank you for purchasing this book and I genuinely hope you get a lot of use and understanding from it. I believe that through our combined actions and by increasing our awareness and knowledge, we can reduce the epidemics we are facing in healthcare today.

Disclaimers

Medical Establishments: As mentioned in the introduction, this is not a book to fight against the medical establishments. You should always seek medical advice. Always get diagnosis from a trained doctor or healthcare professional who is qualified to do so and be sure to talk to your doctor about your plans before implementing them, especially those who are already on medication and under medical care.

Medical Treatment: This book is not supposed to replace good medical treatment and we are not promoting 'cures' for your diseases. The author of this book is not a medical doctor and this is not professional medical advice.

Supplements: When we refer to taking supplements in this book, it is always advisable to talk to your doctor about adding these into your daily diet and routine, especially if you are on medications already.

Just as a side note, when choosing supplements, it is best to find ones that do not have added fillers and that are GMO free. You can always determine this by reading the ingredients.

Filtered Water: Finally, when we refer to fresh and filtered water, we are not referring to distilled water. Distilled water is actually not good for the body because it is essentially 'dead water', meaning that all of the minerals have been taken out of it. When it enters into the body it leeches out all of the minerals from your body and essentially releases them when you go to the toilet.

Prolonged use of distilled water can leave you with a mineral deficiency which will cause you a lot of other issues.

So when we talk about filtered water, we are not talking about distilled water, or bottled water (as the plastic can be toxic and seep into the water especially when left in hot areas), or tap water (as there are many chemicals found in tap water). We are talking about water that has gone through a 'Reverse Osmosis' filter or something like a 'Brita Filter'. These are the best types to use.

If you are going somewhere and want water, put the filtered water into a BPA free plastic bottle (BPA is a harmful chemical found in plastics) or in a copper jug or metal flask.

Ok, let's get into this!

Understanding The Epidemic

So, what are these epidemics we are facing today? Where do they stem from?

In this section we will look at some of the correlations between disease rates and the increases in a range of factors that could be causing them.

Now, correlation does not always equal causation, but we shall let you be the judge of that in this case.

There is strong evidence now that not only do these things seem to correlate but when we explore the potential causes a little more it becomes clear that they could indeed be causing the problems.

So, what exactly is the epidemic we are facing?

Quite simply put it is the absolute explosion of a range of diseases at the same time like we have never seen before in the history of the modern world.

In the last 20 – 25 years, as you will see, these conditions have just started to sky rocket within the society, especially western society.

Here are some of the statistics

Cancer UK
- In the UK there is an estimated total of 2.5million people diagnosed with cancer, which will rise to 4million by 2030. A rise of around

half a million people over the last 5 years (2010
– 2015) - Macmillan
-   By the end of 2016, the people diagnosed with
    cancer will reach 1,000 a day - Macmillan
-   An estimated 162,000 people die from cancer
    every year – Macmillan

This is actual diagnosed cases, the estimated life time
risk of developing cancer is around 1 in 3 people.

Diabetes UK
-   In the UK in 2014 the estimated number of
    people who had been diagnosed with diabetes
    was 3.2million – diabetes.co.uk
-   This is estimated to rise by 5 million by 2025 –
    diabetes.co.uk
-   There is an estimated 24,000 diabetes related
    deaths each year – NHS

**Dementia UK (in this book we address
Alzheimer's the most common form of dementia)**
-   In 2015 there is as estimated 850,000 people
    with dementia – Alzheimers.org.uk
-   By 2025 this will have risen to over 1million
    people – Alzheimers.org.uk
-   There are an estimated 60,000 dementia
    related deaths each year – Alzheimers.org.uk

**Autoimmune Disease UK (let us just look at
Rheumatoid Arthritis, Celiac Disease,
Fibromyalgia and MS)**
-   In the UK, over 400,000 people are affected by
    Rheumatoid Arthritis - NHS
-   An estimated 1 in 100 people are affected by
    Celiac Disease - NHS
-   It is estimated that around 1 in 20 people could

be affected by Fibromyalgia in some way - NHS
-   There is estimated 100,000 people in the UK affected by MS - NHS

This is just 4 of the 80+ autoimmune diseases out there.

Cardiovascular Disease UK (Heart and Circulatory Disease)
-   An estimated 7million people are living with some form of cardiovascular disease – British Heart Foundation
-   An estimated 160,000 people die from a cardiovascular related disease each year – British Heart Foundation

Cancer US
-   In 2015 alone, the number of people diagnosed with cancer is estimated to be 1.6million with an estimated 590,000 deaths – cancer.org

This is again based on actual diagnosed cases, the estimated lifetime risk is about the same as the UK, at 1 in 3 people.

Diabetes US
-   In 2015 an estimated 21million people have been diagnosed with diabetes – American Diabetes Association
-   An estimated 4,660 people are diagnosed with diabetes everyday – American Diabetes Association

- There is an estimated 69,000 diabetes related deaths each year – American Diabetes Association

Dementia US (in this book we address Alzheimer's the most common form of dementia)
- In 2015 there is an estimated 5.3 million people with Dementia – Alzheimer's Association
- In 2015 there is an estimated 700,000 dementia related deaths – Alzheimer's Association

Autoimmune Disease US (let us just look at Rheumatoid Arthritis, Celiac Disease, Fibromyalgia and MS)
- There are an estimated 50million people with some form of autoimmune disease - American Autoimmune Related Diseases Association
- About 1.3million Americans have Rheumatoid Arthritis – healthline.com
- An estimated 1 in 133 Americans have Celiac Disease – CeliacCentral.org
- Approximately 1 in 50 Americans have Fibromyalgia – MyFibro.com
- An estimated 400,000 people have MS, with 200 new cases diagnosed each week – healthline.com

Again, this is just 4 of the 80+ autoimmune diseases out there.

Cardiovascular Disease US (Heart and Circulatory Disease)
- An estimated 85.6million people are living with some form of cardiovascular disease –

heart.org
- Around 2,150 people die every day from a cardiovascular related condition – heart.org

These are just some of the problems we are facing and that we are going to address in this book. As you can see, this is a growing problem and estimates for the future see these figures continuing to rise.

Below we will look at some of the graphs that represent the rise of these diseases and the possible causes of them.

Before we do that though there are some overarching factors that seem to be a theme:

- GMO foods and strong harmful pesticides began to be introduced to the food chain in around the mid 1980's to the mid 1990's and continues to this day.

- The western diet has been increasing in the amount of processed, fatty and sugary foods that are consumed.

- The number of vaccines given to children under 6 years of age has also more than doubled between the early 1980's and 2013.

- Since the late 1980's there has been an increase across the board of a wide range of diseases and conditions, especially in younger children and young adults like never seen before in the West.

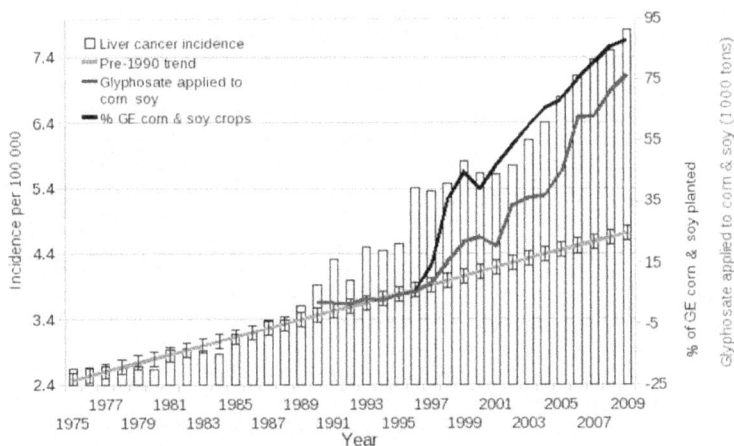

Temporal trends for autism in the USA and the UK

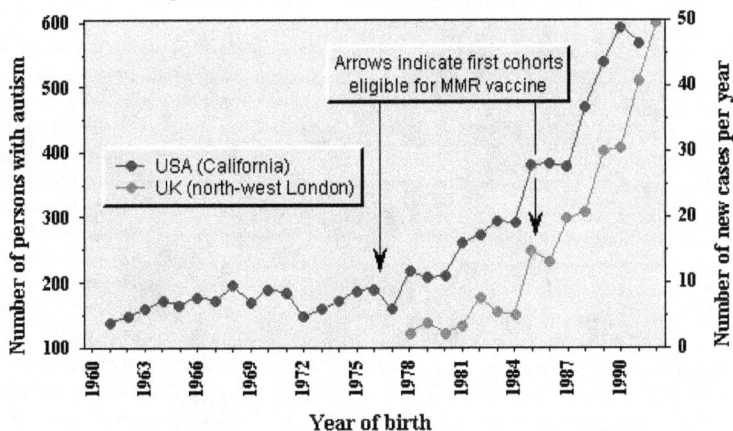

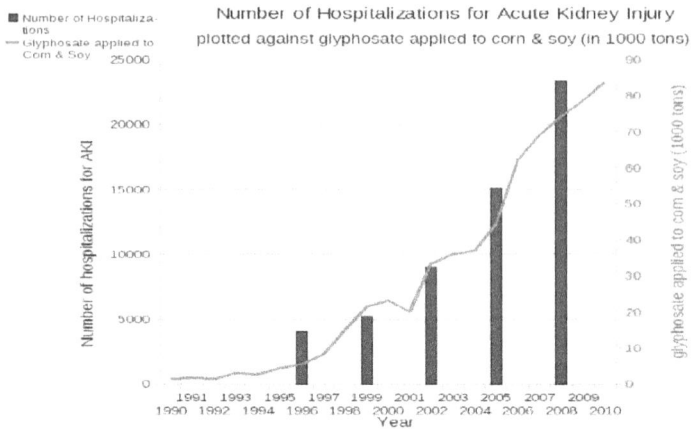

Number of Hospitalizations for Acute Kidney Injury
plotted against glyphosate applied to corn & soy (in 1000 tons)

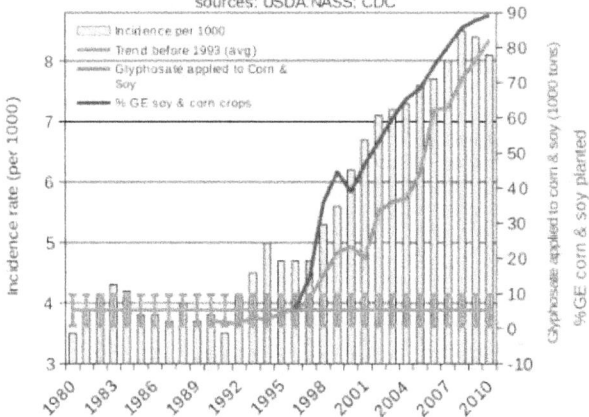

Annual Incidence of Diabetes (age adjusted)

plotted against %GE corn & soy crops planted (R = 0.9547, p <= 1.978e-06)
along with glyphosate applied to corn & soy in US (R = 0.935, p <= 8.303e-08)
sources: USDA NASS; CDC

Figure 14. Correlation between age-adjusted diabetes incidence and glyphosate applications
and percentage of US corn and soy crops that are GE.

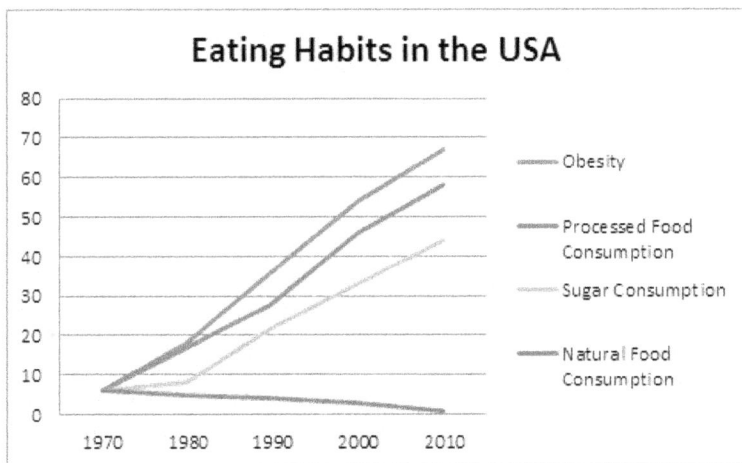

Eating Habits in the USA

- Obesity
- Processed Food Consumption
- Sugar Consumption
- Natural Food Consumption

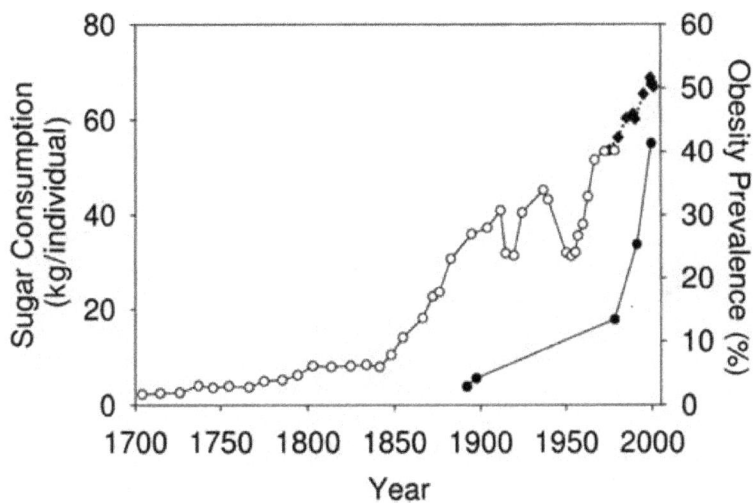

25

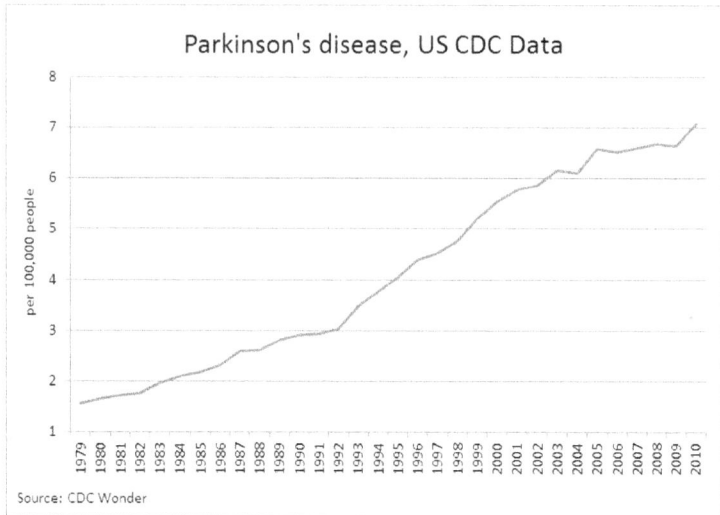

Parkinson's disease, US CDC Data

Source: CDC Wonder

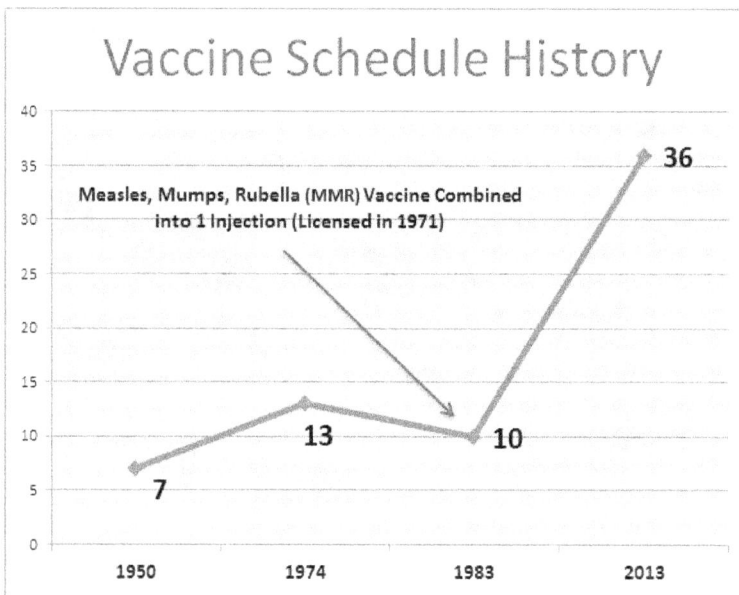

Vaccine Schedule History

Measles, Mumps, Rubella (MMR) Vaccine Combined into 1 Injection (Licensed in 1971)

As you can see from the statistics, a lot of things have

been introduced into our lives that weren't there in those amounts or at all prior to the 1980's.

Could this be the cause of the epidemic we are facing? GMO foods, harmful pesticides, chemicals being inserted into us via vaccines, sugar consumption and processed foods?

Now remember, correlation does not always equal causation. If it did, judging by the graphs below we could also say that an increase in sugar consumption increases life expectancy and that bottled water is what has led to the obesity epidemic...

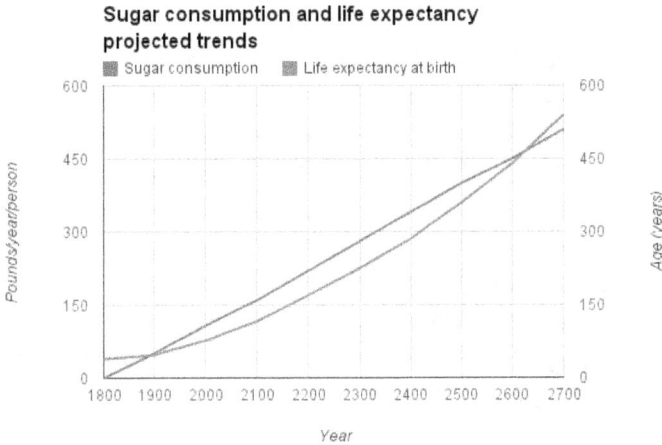

Sugar consumption and life expectancy projected trends

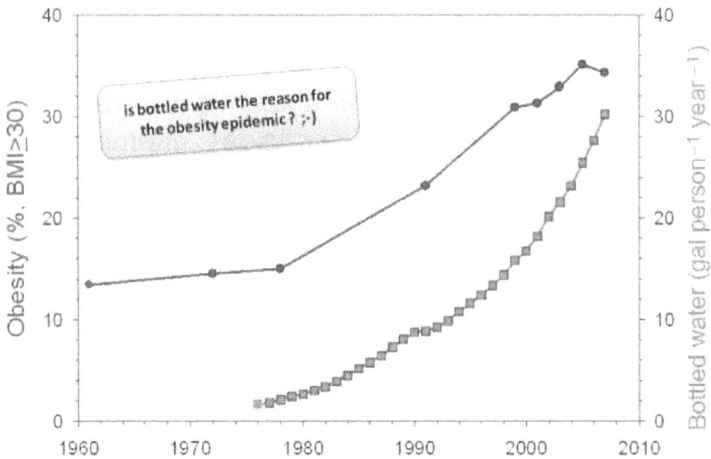

So I'm not concluding anything here. But judge for yourself and look into each of the mentioned areas (GMOs, processed foods, chemicals in vaccines and the vaccines themselves (and neurotoxins) and sugars effect on the body) and come to your own conclusions.

One thing is certain though... There has definitely been a change in the last 20 - 25 years or so that has led to a huge increase in the diseases we are now seeing rising in western society.

Let's look at some of the facts surrounding some of the topics we just mentioned.

- GMOS

So, what is a GMO?
GMO stands for Genetically Modified Organism. This

essentially means that the original plant in question, for example some corn, has been mixed with the genes of something else, like a bacteria or another plant, in order to give it some new desirable trait.

There are two main types of GM crops today.

- The type that is modified to produce its own pesticide from within every cell of the plant as to stop bugs from eating it.

- The type that is modified to be able to withstand and live through large amounts of harmful herbicide being sprayed on it that kills all other weeds around the plant.

What is the aim of GM crops?

The idea and purpose behind the creation of GM crops was to increase yields of the plants grown, stop bugs from eating the growing crops whilst reducing the amount of pesticide needed to be sprayed on crops and having the potential to feed the millions of hungry people the world over with good, nutritional food.

What is the potential problem with GM foods?

While in theory GM crops sound very good, the reality is that the outcome has not been promising so far.

The main problems at the moment seem to be that:

- The actual act of mixing the genes to get the desired trait in a plant is creating unforeseen proteins during that process that are toxic and allergenic.

- The powerful chemical herbicides used to spray on the modified crops are staying there and when consumed are actually quite harmful to our gut biome and body [which as we will see later, the gut is of very high important in our overall health].

There are many independent studies coming forward now with information stating that 'Glyphosate' [also known as 'round-up' herbicide made by the largest GMO manufacturer, Monsanto] may be:

- Contributing to the enhanced growth of harmful pathogenic bacteria's in the environment

- Not as biodegradable as first thought and is found in water supplies, food and the air

- It has been classed as a 'probable carcinogenic' by the World Health Organisation

- A 'Chelator' which means it takes in micronutrient metals like manganese and magnesium, which are vital to the body, but does not release them back out and so depletes the system of it

- Causing bacteria to become resistant to antibiotics

There are also many, many independent studies coming forth now about the affect the GM crops and Glyphosate are having on the biology of animals that have been subjected to these foods. Here are just a few:

- A chronic toxicity study out of Egypt by a Dr. Oraby on albino rats with a range of combined parameters such as biochemical, histopathological and cytogenic to evaluate the negative impact of a GM diet on animals.

  They concluded that the results indicated that there are health hazards linked to the ingestion of diets containing genetically modified components through a range of biochemical alterations, increased number of germ cells with chromosomal abnormalities and fragmented DNA in liver cells.

- A group led by Dr. Kruger looked into dairy cows from 8 separate dairy farms in Denmark fed with GM crops.

  The urine was tested and all were found to be positive for Glyphosate and all had very low levels of the essential minerals manganese and copper in the system that are essential and perform a wide range of important tasks.

  This result has also been echoed by many other studies into the chelation effects of Glyphosate too.

There are many more studies out there, so please do go and look into some of them and come to your own conclusions.

Important to know

I think it is very important to note here that GMO food is literally in all processed foods in the US. In Europe, whilst the direct selling of foods containing GMOs is not allowed anymore, but was when it first came about, GMOs are allowed to be fed to animals for feed.

This essentially means that meat that is not organic and grass fed will still have GMOs within it and then will enter into your system that way and milk that is not from grass fed organic cattle will also have the same.

- Vaccines

What is a vaccine?

A vaccine is a compound that is designed to stimulate an immune response to a specific infectious agent.

The reason for this is so that when the person given the vaccine does actually come into contact with the infectious agent, whether it be a bacteria or virus, the immune system is already prepared for it and it can mount a quicker response than otherwise.

What is the potential problem with vaccines?

The core idea and premise behind vaccines is a good one, but it may be the execution, amount and additional ingredients of the vaccine that is the problem.

As a vaccine is injected, it essentially gets to bypass the immune system before entering the blood stream.

This is generally because most vaccines, if ingested, would be destroyed and rendered useless.

The problem with this is twofold:

- Most viruses are not contracted by entering straight into the blood stream. They generally will naturally come into contact with the immune system first in some way.

When there are toxic chemicals in the blood stream, the risk of nerve and tissue damage increases.

- Vaccines do not just contain the active ingredient that aims to stimulate the response. They come with a wide range of other chemical ingredients that also enter straight into the bloodstream and that the body has to deal with.

As we will see further on in this section in the 'So, what have we not been told?' part, a few experts and industry professionals in the field have some interesting things to say about them.

- Processed Foods

What is a processed food?
A processed food is essentially a food that has been altered from its natural whole state. This can include a

wide range of foods from breakfast cereals right up to the obvious crisps, hamburgers, fizzy drinks and other junk foods we see today.

What is the problem with processed foods?

I think most people would agree that junk food is not good for their health?

This is because junk food is generally devoid of fibre and most of the micro-nutrients the body needs. It contains high amounts of salt, refined sugars, fats, additives and emulsifiers that do not do the body any good at all and actually contribute to the damage and deterioration of the body.

Essentially, the body was not designed to consume this type of food and in today's society people are eating very high amounts of these processed foods. The body was designed to consume whole, natural and nutrient rich foods.

As we mentioned, processed foods also includes things like cereal too. Millions of people start every day with a breakfast cereal because they believe it to be a healthy choice, but this too is a processed food that generally has high levels of added sugars, even the cereals touted as 'healthy', but especially the ones aimed at children and as you will see in the next section 'Sugar Consumption', this is not a good thing.

Sugar Consumption

Sugar consumption is a real concern today. As we mentioned above, literally all processed foods contain added sugar and refined sugars as this is one of the main factors that actually drives the taste and the continued consumption of processed foods amongst consumers.

Normal 'sugar' contains glucose and fructose. While the body needs glucose to power the cells, excessive amounts build up in the blood and lead to a range of problems such as weight gain (as we will see in the 'Obesity' section of the book), diabetes (which we have talked about in the 'Diabetes (Type 2)' section of the book) and can also lead to hardening of the arteries called 'Atherosclerosis' (which we will see in the 'Cardiovascular Disease' section of the book).

The other problem is that fructose is metabolised in a different way to glucose. Fructose goes straight to the liver where, in excessive amounts, turns to fat which can cause the condition 'fatty liver'. This can damage and block the proper functioning of the liver which is a very important organ in the body for a wide range of processes and thus associated serious problems can occur.

You may be thinking *'but fructose is the main sugar in fruits?'* and you would be right, but when you get fructose from fruit it also comes with a range of other health benefits, such as fibre, vitamins and antioxidants that the body needs. Fructose is stored in the liver for later energy use. Here we are talking about excessive amounts and if you consume it from extracted sugar or refined sugars, you are more than likely consuming it in excess.

As well as adding fat to the liver, a high sugar diet will also add fat around the abdomen, kidneys and intestines which can then cause issues stemming from these areas not functioning properly due to congestion and blockages.

Sugar in this form actually has no nutritional value and it is also very addictive. Sugar stimulates the reward centres of the brain, the dopamine receptors, and as such is like a drug as drugs like cocaine also stimulate these centres and work in much the same way.

This is why people who try to come off sugar who have a high sugar diet can find it hard and also have strong cravings for sweet things.

What's more, sugar also feeds a lot of things in the body that we really want to keep down and in check, such as 'Candida' which is present in the gut (see the 'Candida' section for more on that), feeds any harmful parasites that make their way into the gut, fuels cancer growth in those that have it and makes the blood more acidic which in turn leeches the body of its nutrients as it tries to balance out the blood.

This in no way means we are advocating the use of artificial sweeteners as an alternative.

Artificial sweeteners are harmful chemicals that have very negative effects on the working of the whole body, including the nervous system which we will see in the 'Holistic Nervous System Building' section.

So, what have we not been told?
Finally, before we step into the main content of the book, I would just like to include these points from 'whistle blowers' who are those people who have

worked in these industries for many years and have decided to come out with what they have witnessed and done and what really happens behind closed doors that the public generally doesn't get to hear about.

Whistle blower testimonials On GMOs

- Dr. Thierry Vrain is a former soil biologist and genetic scientist who worked for 'Agriculture Canada' (a manufacturer of GMO foods) for 30 years. He was also the spokesperson for the safety of GMO crops there.

  Since retiring and leaving the company, he has continued his scientific research into GM crops that, due to his job, he had not previously looked at.

  He now has switched sides and talks of the dangers of GMO crops. He has said things such as:

  > "It's almost as if the entire population of North America is on a low-grade antibiotic day in, day out from birth, everyday, so this is the reality" [This was when talking about Glyphosate ('Round-Up' Herbicide) a very powerful herbicide used with the GM crops]

  > "I refute the claims of the biotechnology companies that their engineered crops yield more, that they require less

pesticide applications and that they are safe to eat"

"The scientific literature is full of studies showing that engineered corn and soya contain toxic or allergenic proteins" [Which factory farmed animals the world over are fed and then pass onto the people that eat them]

"Engineered food by definition is depleted of metal micronutrients because it contains residues of a strong 'Chelator' [something that holds onto the metal micronutrients and does not give them to the plant]. Your microbiome and gut intestines are, of course, first inline. After a few years of eating depleted food, other organs start to show"

"There are several studies to show that if you eat engineered crops, the bacteria in your intestines who are extremely numerous and do all kinds of useful things, the transgenes [from the altered crops] find their way into the bacteria of the gut. This is documented. There is no argument. This is called 'Lateral Gene Transfer'" [This ultimately means that your gut ecosystem is being changed and altered by these foreign genes]

"In 1996 the research scientists of the FDA predicted that engineered foods would contain rogue proteins that could be toxins, cause allergies and nutritional deficiencies and other diseases. This is documented. This is published. The administration ignored them and went ahead and accepted the crops"

"The proteins are just not what is expected"

"The bio-tech companies grant a great deal of money to universities to do research on their products. Very little about safety testing, but a lot of money goes to universities and most of the publications coming out of that grant money say that the technology is safe and innocuous. Then there is another body of research done by other labs without grants from the bio-tech industry that show exactly the opposite. That the technology is not safe, that the proteins are not safe, that some of them are actually quite allergenic or toxic"

- Kirk Azevedo is a former Monsanto employee [the largest GMO manufacturer in the world]. He quickly left the company after he witnessed a range of careless acts from them with regards to the genetically engineered cotton plants they had fed to cows.

> "I went in there with the idea of helping and healing and came out with 'Oh, I guess it is just another profit-orientated company'"

Kirk recalls that the way they were doing the gene insertion from the bacteria to the plant was very 'messy'. It essentially used a 'gene gun' that bombards the plant tissue with genes and he knew from his previous training that this approach could cause changes and mutations in the DNA which may result in new harmful proteins forming.

"I was afraid at this time that some of these proteins may be toxic"

He was concerned that these rogue proteins could lead to:

"Mad cow or some other prion-type disease"

He attempted to share his concerns with one of the scientists there:

"He had no idea what I was talking about; he had not even heard of prions. This was at a time when Europe had a great concern about mad cow disease"

He then continues:

"So I am explaining to him about the potential untoward effects of these foreign proteins, but he just did not understand"

Kirk became upset with this and complained to the PhD in charge of feeding the experimental plants to the cows.

He explained that unknown proteins that had been created during the gene insertion phase, including prions, might even affect humans who consume the cow's milk and meat. The scientist replied:

"Well that's what we're doing everywhere else and that's what we're doing here"

He refused to destroy the plants.

"I approached pretty much everyone on my team in Monsanto. Once they understood my perspective, I was somewhat ostracised. It seemed as if once I started questioning things, people wanted to keep their distance from me. I lost the cooperation with other team members. Anything that interfered with advancing the commercialisation of this technology was going to be pushed aside"

- Dr Arpad Pusztai is a bio-chemist and nutritionist who spent 30 years at the Rowett Research Institute of Nutrition and Health. He is also an expert on plant lectins who has authored 270 papers and 3 books on the subject.

Dr Pusztai pointed out that substances in GM foods that have a slow acting affect would not be detected in the short term studies that these bio companies currently do.

In his own studies he noted that rats developed immune system defects and stunted growth after a time period that corresponds to about 10 human years.

He was one of the first to speak out about GM foods in 1998 when he said publicly that he would not eat GM foods. He was ridiculed, suspended from his 30 year position and made an outcast by the bio-tech companies and scientists in the media. Since then, many more scientists have come forward with the same findings as Dr Pusztai.

> "The main problem with this GM food business is that GM foods, that is GM soya and GM corn, were introduced sort of 'under the counter'. By the time this broadcast went out [the one in 1998 mentioned above] it was about 15 – 18 months that the British public were eating this stuff without knowing. They just kept very quiet about it"

> "To give you an idea, 3 years into the program we were the only people that did this job and it took 3 years for us to realise that the public are eating this stuff. Even we didn't know it"

> "I think they tried to make it such that

there would be no problem or reaction by the consumers"

"We had been doing this research, we were 3 years well into it, and I started out, and most of the team started out, that this is a great idea. Then we started to get the results and the results did tell us otherwise, that there are problems and that these problems ought to be addressed rather than swept under the carpet"

Whistle blower testimonials On Vaccines

- Dr. William Thompson a former Senior Scientist with the Centers for Disease Control (CDC) came out with this statement recently:

  "I regret that my co-authors and I omitted statistically significant information in our 2004 article published in the 'Journal of Paediatrics'. The omitted data suggested that African American males who received the MMR vaccine before age 36 months were at increased risk for autism. Decisions were made regarding which findings to report after the data were collected, and I believe the final study protocol was not followed".

  "I cannot believe we did what we did, but we did"

"It's the lowest point of my career that I went along with that paper".

In reply to this, Scientist Dr. David Lewis a research microbiologist and an international expert in whistleblowing and the detection of scientific fraud reviewed the original CDC documents and then the paper they published in 2004, and had this to say:

"Probably this is the clearest case and easiest case in which to answer is it fraud or is it an accident. Clearly it is fraud".

- Dr. Theresa Deisher is a PhD graduate in Molecular and Cellular Physiology from Stanford University and has worked in the bio-technology field for over 19 years.

She is also the founder of:

  o AVM Biotechnology [a company that develops and commercialises 'safe, effective and ethical stem cell technologies for regenerative medicine, oncology and fully human biologics']

  o Sound Choice Pharmaceutical Institute [a company founded to 'promote consumer awareness about the widespread use of electively aborted fetal material in drug discovery, development and commercialisation']

Dr. Deisher actually testified at the 'Minnesota House HHS Committee' with regards to the links between vaccine use, in particular the MMR vaccine, and Autism and the data they had collected over the past several years.

She testified the following:

> "Firstly, even in the publications that claim no link between MMR and Autism there is an evident Autism change point in 1988.
>
> The authors dismiss the link between Autism and the MMR vaccine because, as they point out, vaccine compliance was well over 95% in the UK before 1988. However, what the authors documented on page 4 at the top right, which is appendix L of our binders [addressing the committee], but failed to investigate was that the MMR vaccine used in the UK was switched in 1988 and 1989. Prior to 1988 the MMR in the UK was produced in animal cell lines and in 1988 and 1989 three new MMRs replaced that original MMR all of which used fetal cell lines for at least one of the viruses contained in the MMR.
>
> Having worked in commercial bio-technology and clinical development programs I was aware of the residuals that would be found in vaccines and having also worked with homologous

recombination and molecular biology I was also aware that the human fetal DNA introduced in vaccines has the potential to illicit auto immune responses or to incorporate into the recipients own genes and disrupt normal protein production"

"What we have found is that across continents and across decades changes in Autism disorder, not considering Autism spectrum, but only Autism disorder, are clearly associated with the introduction of vaccines produced using human fetal cell lines"

- Dr. Shiv Chopra is a microbiologist and human rights activist. He is a former employee of Health Canada for 35 years where he was the Senior Scientific Advisor for the regulatory assessment of food and drugs, including new vaccines.

  He was also the cause for ensuring Monsanto's Bovine Growth Hormone was not approved for use in Canada.

    "The latest figure from the CDC, they say it [the flu shot] is effective in 23% of people"

    "The fact is that the virus [flu virus] always mutates and so we are always taking previous years or from somewhere in the pasts vaccine. So that vaccine doesn't work. If the concern is that the virus in mutating, it takes at least 6 months to take that virus strain and try and make the vaccine. They do not know how the virus has or will mutate beforehand. By the time you have the vaccine for the strain just past, next year is coming around and it will have mutated already to the next strain. So what is the purpose? It doesn't make any sense"

"They are actually creating patients for life from very early childhood by giving vaccines and then wrong foods so that from cradle to grave people will remain patients. The second assault then comes from the drugs and devises [to manage their diseases]. It is big business for the corporations"

- Michelle Rowton is with 'Nurses Against Mandatory Vaccines'. She is a neo-natal nurse practitioner with board certification and certified in neo-natal paediatric support. She has a master of science in nursing (MSc), is a certified registered nurse and has a nursing interventions certification.

She says:

"I think we are giving them [vaccines] too young. I think we are doing way too many at once if we just look at how fast the schedule has grown but I think what a lot of people don't realise is that in a closed space like the NICU [Neo-natal Intensive Care Unit] is that they have decided we need to vaccinate these babies on time. 2 months after they are born... bam, there it goes. This baby could be 4 months early and still supposed to be inside their mother and weighing 3 or 4 pounds and are given the same amount of vaccine as a 200 pound man and I've sat in a room with our on call staff physicians and practitioners [with them saying] 'oh wow, this is so embarrassing, this 25 weeker never actually required a breathing tube and going on the vent after he was born because he was so strong, but we gave him his 2 month vaccination and he got intubated last night' like it's funny"

"The step down units are calling the NICU saying 'hey, were going to go ahead and give these 4 babies their 2 month shot today, make sure you have beds ready' because we all know their going to have increased breathing difficulties, feeding and digesting difficulties, apnoea [forgetting to breath] and bradycardia [abnormally slow heart action]. This is what goes on"

A study that followed this from JAMA Paediatrics [The Journal of the American Medical Association] confirmed that extremely low birth weight [ELBW] infants in the NICU had increased incidence of sepsis evaluations and increased respiratory support and intubation after routine immunisation.

- Marcia Angell is the former editor for 20 years of the 'New England Journal of Medicine' which is one of the most prestigious medical journals out there. She had this to say about pharmaceuticals:

> "It is simply no longer possible to believe much clinical research that is published, or to reply on the judgement of trusted physicians or authoritative medical guidelines. I take no pleasure in this conclusion, which I reached slowly over my two decades as an editor of the 'New England Journal of Medicine'".

> "No one knows the total amount [of money] provided by drug companies to physicians, but I estimate from the annual reports of the top 9 U.S based drug companies that it comes to tens of billions of dollars a year in North America alone. By such means, the pharmaceutical industry has gained enormous control over how doctors evaluate and use its own products. Its extensive ties to physicians, particularly senior faculty at prestigious medical schools, affect the results of research, the way medicine is practiced, and even the definition of what constitutes a disease".

- Finally, Dr Mark Randall (who uses that name to protect his identity and risk of harassment and loss of his pension) is said to be a former vaccine researcher and maker and worked for the Nation Institute of Health (NIH). He is also said to have worked in the labs of a range of pharmaceutical companies too.

Note: While this comes from an anonymous source as it's under a fake name and so cannot be 100% verified, we thought it would be note-worthy to include here as it echoes what a lot of other independent professionals have said with regards to this topic:

> "On a scientific level, people need information, so that they can choose well. It is one thing to say choice is good, but if the atmosphere is full of lies, how can you choose? Also, if the FDA [Food and Drug Administration] were run by honourable people, these vaccines would not be granted licenses. They would be investigated to within an inch of their lives"

In a question that stated 'There are medical historians who state that the overall decline of illnesses was not due to vaccines' he replied:

> "I know. For a long time, I ignored their work"

> "Because I was afraid of what I would find out. I was in the business of

50

developing vaccines. My livelihood depended on continuing that work"

He then went on to say:

"I did my own investigations. The decline of disease is due to improved living conditions, cleaner water, advanced sewage systems, nutrition, fresher food, a decrease in poverty. Germs may be everywhere, but when you are healthy, you don't contract the diseases as easily"

He was then asked 'what did you feel when you completed your own investigations'

"Despair. I realised I was working in a sector based on a collection of lies"

"They [vaccines] involve the human immune system in a process that tends to compromise immunity. They can actually cause the disease they are supposed to prevent"

All of this info comes from industry professionals who have been working closely in these areas and there is a lot more out there too.

The purpose of displaying this information was to just allow you to see that there can be hidden motives within these multi-billion pound, profit driven companies when it comes to health.

This is not to say you should distrust all corporations, medical institutions and doctors, but just to open up the avenues of exploration for you and to allow you to see that there are two sides to the story we are given.

I implore you to seriously look into these areas that we have talked about in this section of the book and start to really dig into the independent research, cover-ups, intentions and possible motives behind these multi-billion pound corporations and make your own judgements about what is going on.

Being told what to think is never a good way to live your life, and that includes from this book.

The best way is to sincerely look into all aspects of something and then come to an educated conclusion of how you can personally proceed. After all, it is your life to lead and nobody else's.

Ok, so now we have gone over the background information and given the book some context, we can now begin our journey of understanding the body and looking at the solutions to the problems we are facing today.

The Body Essentials

First and foremost, lets start with the essentials the body needs.

The human body needs a range of nutrients in order for it to function correctly. There is a category of 'essential' nutrients within that list that the body must receive from outside sources and are, well essential, for the processes of the system and so we must have them if we want to have optimal health.

There are two main categories of nutrients. These are macro nutrients and micro nutrients.

Macro nutrients are:

- Proteins (Amino acids)
- Carbohydrates
- Fats

Micro nutrients are:

- Vitamins
- Minerals

Below we have listed both these macro and micro essential nutrients and, at the end, have included the foods that should be consumed to ensure you get all of these. The categories are proteins (amino acids), fats, carbohydrates, vitamins and minerals.

Protein (Amino Acids)
There are 20 amino acids that the body uses to create

all of the proteins in the system. Proteins are not just something we consume to build muscle. Proteins are essential for the creation and production of enzymes and some hormones, catalytic processes in the body, they carry oxygen and other nutrients around in the blood stream, make up all the connective tissues and help the muscles to contract. They are fundamental to life.

The body does not absorb proteins though. Instead it breaks them down into the individual amino acids, absorbs these and then these amino acids can be reassembled into other proteins to do the job that is needed.

All of the thousands of different types of proteins though are made from these 20 amino acids.

Out of these 20 amino acids, there are 10 essential ones and 10 that can be synthesised within the body. So really only 10 have to be brought in from an outside source.

The 10 Essential Amino Acids

1. Arginine
2. Histidine
3. Isoleucine
4. Leucine
5. Lysine
6. Methionine
7. Phenylalanine
8. Threonine
9. Tryptophan
10. Valine

You can go down to the 'Foods containing the amino acids, fats, carbohydrates, minerals and vitamins the body needs' section to see what sources you can obtain these from.

Fats

Fats are important in the body and all play a role. They come in three forms:

- **Saturated**

  Saturated fats are the most stable of all the fats. Saturated means the carbon atoms are saturated with hydrogen atoms, meaning there is no space for further atoms to attach.

  When they are heated to high temperatures they do not degrade and go rancid. This is good because fats that degrade produce harmful by-product oxides which damage the body.

  Saturated fat is needed for the proper functioning and health of all the cell membranes and the 'myelin' that covers the nerves. Contrary to popular belief, you do indeed need saturated fats in your diet.

  The healthiest form of saturated fat is coconut oil and can provide more than is necessary for your saturated fat needs.

- **Monounsaturated**

  Monounsaturated fats are the second most stable. So when they are heated to high temperatures they only slightly degrade and go

55

rancid.

Monounsaturated fats come in the form of fruit oils like olive and avocado. For this reason, it is always best to get 'cold pressed' oils.

They are very useful for keeping the circulatory system healthy.

- **Polyunsaturated**
Polyunsaturated fats are the most unstable of the three and have multiple 'gaps' and available carbon atoms.

When they are heated to high temperatures they degrade much more, go rancid and turn into oxidation products which give off harmful by-products that damage the cells, tissues and gut.

These are generally the vegetable oils such as soy, corn and canola oils.

While highly unstable, the essential omega-3 fatty acids are actually polyunsaturated and, just like saturated fats, are essential to the body.

- o Omega 3 fatty acids (ALA, EPA and DHA)
  - Flax and Chia Seeds (ground) – good sources of ALA (ground chia seeds also slightly raise EPA)
  - Fish Oil and Krill Oil – good sources of EPA and DHA

- Kelp (Wakame) – good sources of EPA
- Algae Oils – good sources of DHA

- **Trans fats and hydrogenated oils**
It was because of the highly reactive state of polyunsaturated fats that hydrogenation and trans fats actually came about.

In order to try and make the vegetable oils more stable, they were put through the process of hydrogenation. This is when the oils are hardened in order to make them less reactive (as unsaturated fats stay liquid at room temperature while saturated fats solidify).

The problem with this is that it created what is known as 'trans fats'.

Trans fats are modified fats and as such are actually harmful and toxic to the system and interrupt with the normal health of cell membranes. They are also now present in most processed and junk foods as most of them use these kinds of oils.

Saturated fat is not the bad fat... trans fat is.

The omega 3's and saturated fats are needed across the body for processes such as adding permeability to the cell membrane, governing the signals that go in and out of the cells, healthy brain function and healthy joints.

They are also used as a precursor to some hormones

being produced in the body and so because of these reasons are very important in the healthy functioning of the body as a whole.

Finally, fats also help with body temperature regulation.

Carbohydrates
Carbohydrates are essentially used in the body to provide energy.

When carbs are broken down in the body they provide energy to the muscles for contracting and other such functions, give fuel to the nervous system and cells and prevents protein from getting broken down for energy.

This then allow for other biological work to take place in the system.

Vitamins
Next up, we have the vitamins. Pretty much all of the vitamins must be obtained from an external source and so we will address all of them.

There are two main classes of vitamins. There are the fat soluble vitamins and then the water soluble vitamins.

Essentially, the difference between the two is this.

Fat soluble vitamins are stored in fats and so stay in the body for longer and because of this it is possible that they can cause toxicity in the body if consumed very often in high amounts and on the other end of the scale if your fat intake or absorption is compromised, then you may become deficient in these vitamins too. The vitamins that are fat soluble are Vitamin A, D, E and K.

Water soluble vitamins, the B vitamins and Vitamin C, are not stored in the body for long periods and are passed through the body easily and so daily intake of them is much more important.

Vitamins are used for a wide range of purposes as you will see below. So we have:

- **Vitamin A**
  Vitamin A is used for bone building, vision, skin, immune system functioning and has antioxidant effects.

- **The B Vitamins (all help to convert carbohydrates into energy):**

  o **Vitamin B1 (Thiamine)**
    B1 is used for keeping the nervous system healthy and improving cardiovascular functioning. It is also needed for hydrochloric acid production

  o **Vitamin B2 (Riboflavin)**
    Helps with production of cellular energy, helps with the processing of amino acids and fats, helps protect the eyes and also acts as an antioxidant

  o **Vitamin B3 (Niacin)**

Helps with digestion, reduces LDL cholesterol build up, helps with hormone production and enzyme activation

- o **Vitamin B4 (Choline)**
  Used as a precursor to other B vitamin assimilation, creation of neurotransmitters, cell membrane health, healthy nervous system and liver function

- o **Vitamin B5 (Pantothenic Acid)**
  Important for enzyme synthesis, adrenal functioning, stimulates metabolism, an antioxidant and used to keep hair healthy

- o **Vitamin B6**
  Required for production of insulin, production of red and white blood cells, healthy nerves and muscles and creation of DNA and RNA

- o **Vitamin B7**
  Used in the regulation of glucose and amino acids and keeps the nails and hair healthy

- o **Vitamin B9 (Folate)**
  Helps to control cholesterol, cardiovascular health, health of muscle tissues and is important in the formation of red blood cells

- o **Vitamin B12**
  Aids in the production of red blood cells,

maintains the health of the central nervous system and its protective lining and the production and maintenance of DNA and RNA

- **Vitamin C**
Vitamin C is a powerful antioxidant for the body and is also important for maintaining the lining of the arteries and blood vessel. It is also important for the growth and repair of tissues in every part of the body, helps to produce collagen which is important for skin and connective tissues, helps with healing wounds and healing and maintaining bones and teeth.

- **Vitamin D**
Vitamin D is used for the healthy functioning of all cells, calcium absorption and switching genes on and off. It strengthens and maintains the immune system, nervous system, bones, joints and muscles, helps to reduce swelling and inflammation and helps to control blood pressure and blood sugar.

- **Vitamin E**
Vitamin E is also a powerful antioxidant and helps to stabilise the cell membranes and protect the cells. It also protects the nervous system and helps to keep the skin strong and healthy too.

- **Vitamin K**

Vitamin K is important for blood clotting and healthy bone formation. It also helps to prevent calcification of the arteries and other tissues in the body and plays a role in blood sugar regulation.

Minerals

The body also utilises a wide range of minerals for a wide range of processes in the system. Here we have listed the essential minerals that must be obtained from an external source with a brief explanation as to the important roles they play.

They come in two forms. 'Macro minerals' and 'Trace minerals'.

Macro minerals:

- **Calcium**
  Calcium is important for bone formation, cell processes, muscle contraction and blood clotting.

- **Magnesium**
  Magnesium is important for nerve impulses, enzyme activation and protein synthesis.

- **Phosphorus**
  Phosphorus is important for bone and teeth structure, cell membrane formation, the workings of inside the cell and pH regulation.

- **Sodium**
  Sodium is important for water, pH and

electrolyte regulation, nerve transmission, muscle contraction and hydrochloric acid creation.

- **Chloride**
Chloride is important for pH balance, enzyme activation and hydrochloric acid creation.

- **Potassium**
Potassium is important for maintaining water balance in the body, electrolyte and pH regulation and cell membrane transfer.

Trace minerals:

- **Chromium**
Chromium is an important trace mineral for helping insulin to do its job and get glucose into the cells effectively.

- **Cobalt**
Cobalt is an important trace mineral that is essential for the formation of vitamin b12 which, as we mentioned, is important for red blood cell creation and keeping the nervous system healthy and functioning correctly.

- **Copper**
Copper is an important trace mineral that plays major roles in breaking down nutrients, creation of neurotransmitters, pigment formation, strengthening connective tissue, nervous system development and important for enzyme creation.

- **Iodine**

Iodine is an important trace mineral that is essential for thyroid function, healthy metabolism of cells, neurological cell development, fetal development and much more.

- **Iron**
Iron is an important trace mineral that is essential for the transportation of oxygen around the body and removal of carbon dioxide, production of red blood cells, converting blood sugar to energy, enzyme production, healthy immune system, physical and mental growth and more.

- **Manganese**
Manganese is an important trace mineral that is essential for a healthy liver, kidney and pancreas. It helps to form connective tissue, bones, helps the blood to clot properly, the production of sex hormones, fat and carbohydrate metabolism, blood sugar regulation and calcium absorption.

- **Selenium**
Selenium is an important trace mineral that is a precursor to the most powerful antioxidant in the body, which is 'Glutathione' which helps to protect against free radical damage to cells and tissues and helps to detox the body of any heavy metal exposure. It is very important for immune function and health.

- **Zinc**
Zinc is an important trace mineral for a wide range of things such as enzyme and hormone

creation, immune health and functioning, connective tissues, muscle growth, artery health, eye health, hydrochloric acid production and reproductive organ health and functioning.

- **Molybdenum**
  Molybdenum is an important trace element for enzyme activation, helps with the breakdown of nutrients into useable forms, helps with production of energy within the core of the cell and a range of other processes in the body.

One very important thing we must take into consideration with minerals and that would be advisable for you to remember as we go through this book is that in plant based foods, minerals are obtained from the soils they are grown in.

If the soil is deficient in the minerals, as many conventionally farmed soils are today, then the plant too will be deficient in these minerals and thus we will not get them.

This is why it is important to go organic as much as possible but to also supplement where needed.

This is also true for factory farmed, non-organic or grass fed animals, as they are eating GMO, conventionally grown feeds that will too be deficient in these minerals.

Foods containing the amino acids, fats, carbohydrates, minerals and vitamins the body needs

So here is a list of all the foods that will give the body what it requires if eaten predominantly organic, fresh and raw where possible. Remember, there is also the option of supplementing where needed too.

The foods are:

-   **Protein:** Sesame seeds, pumpkin seeds, sunflower seeds and other seeds, most beans like kidney beans etc, lentils, brown rice and nuts. Animal sources will be meats and dairy.

-   **Fats:** Coconut, olives, avocado, krill oil/algae oil/seaweed/chia/flax (omega'3s), nuts and seeds. Animal sources will again be meats and dairy.

-   **Carbohydrates:** Can be obtained from all types of beans, potatoes, grains, fruits and some vegetables.

-   **Vitamin A:** Sweet potatoes, carrots, squash, dark leafy greens, peppers, mangoes and pumpkin (and other yellow and orange coloured fruits and vegetables). Meats too.

-   **B Vitamins. B1:** Sunflower seeds, oats, lentils, beans. **B2:** Spinach, mushrooms, sesame seeds, asparagus, almonds. **B3:** Brown rice, mushrooms, green peas, peanuts, sunflower seeds, avocado. **B4:** Dark leafy greens, brown rice. **B5:** Mushrooms, avocado, sweet potatoes, lentils, broccoli, sunflower seeds. **B6:** Brown rice, sunflower seeds, pistachios,

bananas, avocado, spinach, peppers. **B7:**
Nuts, oats, walnuts, peanuts, almonds, sweet
potatoes, tomatoes, carrots. **B9:** Beans, lentils,
spinach, asparagus, avocado, broccoli, mango,
oranges. **B12:** Organically grown foods (as
B12 comes from bacteria's in the soil) – if not,
you can supplement and dairy and meats
(again, from organic, grass fed animals).

- **Vitamin C:** Oranges, kale, papaya, bell
  pepper, brussel sprouts, broccoli, pineapple,
  berries, kiwi, guava and many more fruits and
  vegetables.

- **Vitamin D:** The primary source is the sun but
  can also be obtained from dairy and
  supplements (D3).

- **Vitamin E:** Almonds, sunflower seeds, olives,
  pumpkin seeds, sesame seeds, dark leafy
  greens and nuts.

- **Vitamin K:** Dark leafy greens.

- **Minerals. Calcium:** Dark leafy greens, dairy.
  Phosphorus: Pumpkin seeds, squash seeds,
  brazil nuts, beans and lentils. **Magnesium:**
  Dark leafy greens, squash, pumpkin seeds,
  lentils, brown rice, avocado, bananas, dark
  chocolate. **Sulphur:** Garlic, onions, kale,
  broccoli, cauliflower, cabbage, leeks and
  chives. **Sodium/Chloride:** Sea salt.

Potassium: Bananas, dark leafy greens, beans, potatoes, avocado and mushrooms.

- **Trace Minerals. Chromium:** Broccoli, oats, green beans, grapes, sweet potatoes, onions, garlic, beetroot. **Cobalt:** Nuts, dark leafy greens and oats. **Copper:** Sesame seeds, kale, mushrooms, cashews, chickpeas and avocados. **Iodine:** Seaweed, potatoes, himalayan salt, navy beans, cranberries. **Iron:** Dark leafy greens, brown rice, beans, nuts and seeds. **Manganese:** Hazelnuts, seeds, beans, dark leafy greens. **Selenium:** Brazil nuts, seeds, mushrooms, brown rice, oats. **Zinc:** Pumpkin/squash/flax/sesame/watermelon seeds, cashews, raw chocolate, beans, mushrooms, garlic, chickpeas and brown rice.

By putting all of these into use in your daily diet, you will get the full range of nutrients and minerals that your system needs.

Now we will move into the systems of the body. Namely the nervous system and the immune system.

Holistic Nervous System Building

This is probably one of, if not, the most important part of this book. This is also the reason it is put here before we get into the actual conditions.

The Nervous System. The Nervous System is composed of your brain, spinal cord, nerve cells and then branches that come from this and cover the entire body.

It is the core factor in literally all processes. It is everything, the beginning and the end... literally.

It is what allows all parts of the body to work together, sense the outside world, compute and translate that into something meaningful and what allows the body to function and react.

I cannot stress enough that this is the most important part of the human body. Nothing works, functions or exists in the human body without it.

'Paramahansa Yogananda' who was one of a handful of the first yogis from India to come to the West and teach the science of Yoga (which means union) said: *'The spine and the brain are the altars of God'*"(and don't worry for those of you who are not spiritually inclined, this is not a spiritual book). I do though however encourage everyone to look into this great man and his teachings.

The nervous system is the first thing to start developing after conception, even before the heart, which then gives rise to everything else.

It is then the last thing to die as we leave the physical body, which is why I said it is literally the beginning and the end. The Alpha and The Omega of physical human life.

One more time, and don't worry you will get used to me repeating myself in this book, the nervous system is the most important part of the body and governs all processes. ALL.

Now that is clear, let us talk about how the nervous system is laid out.

The Layout of the Nervous System

Firstly, we have the Central Nervous System (known as the CNS). The CNS is the master controller if you like.

It is located in the brain and the spinal cord. It is so important that it is the only system that is completely encased and protected by bone - the skull and the space in the spine known as the 'vertebral canal'.

Then branching off from this and covering the rest of the body is the Peripheral Nervous System (known as the PNS). This allows the signals from the CNS to be transmitted throughout the rest of the body and allows stimulus to travel back to the CNS from the rest of the body too.

This system of nerves can then be divided into two

main groups:
The Voluntary and Involuntary Nervous System.

The voluntary allows us to control those things that we are conscious of, such as arms, legs, turning our head, jumping up and down, chewing etc.

The Involuntary controls... well everything else. All the millions of processes that continually happen within us without us having to think about it. Hormones, blood flow, pH, breathing (although we can make that conscious as well), growth and all the others. This involuntary system is also better known as the 'Autonomic Nervous System'.

> **This Autonomic Nervous System (ANS)** is then divided again into the Sympathetic and Parasympathetic Nervous Systems. These are the important areas we will be referring to in the book all the time, but don't worry, I will keep reminding you of what they do.

> o **The Sympathetic Nervous System** is what is known as the 'fight or flight' state. Essentially what this means is that it is a type of active state that heightens awareness, moves the blood and energy focus into the extremities and increases processes such as heart rate and blood sugar to, essentially, get the body ready to 'fight' (take on a perceived threat) or 'flight' (run away).

> We name it this because it is probably around the time of early man that this was literally used for these two reasons

in situations of danger and threats from predators.

o **The Parasympathetic Nervous System** is what is known as the 'rest and digest' state. This is the relaxed and calm state which brings focus back into the core of the body to increase blood flow and energy there and as such is conducive to healing, digestion and growth.

So, the Sympathetic Nervous System is the 'fight or flight' state, and the Parasympathetic Nervous System is the 'rest and digest' state.

Why is it important to know this?

It is important to know about these two states because they always come into play when we talk about health and wellbeing.

While it is important for the body to utilise both states in a variety of ways all the time, when the body becomes chronically biased towards the 'fight or flight' state, this poses lots of problems. We call this the stressed state.

The Stressed State
Throughout this book you will see me refer to the sympathetic nervous system state as the 'stressed state'.

Remember, this fight or flight state comes from a primitive time when man had to look out for a lot of dangers and had to react quickly to the world around him in order to literally stay alive.

So, when the fight or flight (or sympathetic nervous system) is activated, cholesterol levels are increased as they are a precursor to stress hormones which are released and lead to a wide range of reactions in the body, such as blood pressure level increasing to pump enough blood to the extremities, blood sugar is elevated to get enough energy to the muscles, energy is used much more quickly, healthy growth is reduced, there is a reduced steroidal output and immunity is also lowered.

All of these come about because the body is focusing on one thing and that is getting out of immediate perceived danger. This is why energy is used quicker, growth slows, steroidal output is reduced and immunity is lowered (because growing, reproducing and protecting you from a disease is not as important as evading that immediate danger).

Even though today most of us do not have these immediate kinds of problems, we still have that primitive part of the brain and response to stressful situations around us. This can also be in the form of emotional stress, physical stress and chemical stress which we will get to in a minute.

In the short run, these changes in processes in the system are not a problem, they evolved in us for a reason, but now the problem comes when we are continually in a stressed state day in day out.

When these reactions and this state is sustained for long periods of time it can turn into things such as:

- Continuously high cholesterol levels, which can lead to plaques forming in the arteries and restrict blood flow

- Continuous high blood pressure which puts a lot of pressure and strain on the arteries and veins and can lead to strokes, heart attacks and other cardiovascular diseases

- High blood sugar which we have extensively explained in the 'Hyperglycaemia' and 'Obesity' sections, but essentially can lead to weight gain, diabetes, cardiovascular diseases, deteriorated arteries and more

- Always low on energy due to the speed at which energy is being used up

- Healthy growth is reduced in areas such as hair, nails and fetal development

- Infertility due to the reduction in steroidal hormones

- Likeliness to get more infections and diseases due to reduced immune response

- Depression and/or anxiety and other neurological disorders due to reduced levels of serotonin and other neurotransmitters

- Bowel problems and digestive issues due to the blood and energy being moved away from the gut into the extremities, which reduces the digestive ability leading to a range of other problems, one of which being nutritional deficiencies

As you can see a wide range of issues comes from being continually in a stressed state.

As I also mentioned, this stressed state can be triggered by emotional stresses, chemical stresses and physical stresses.

- Emotional stresses can include day to day stresses of work life, home life, negative thoughts, being around negative people, low self-esteem, worrying a lot, unsatisfied with life and other things of that nature

- Chemical stresses can include pharmaceutical medications, vaccines, environmental toxins (such as pesticides/herbicides/fungicides, car and other fumes), neurotoxins such as heavy metals in water and other neurotoxins in processed and junk foods and other such exposures to synthetic chemicals in our foods, environments and products.

- Physical stresses can include injuries, damage to the body (externally and internally), burns, pain and other related factors.

It will always be in your best interest to remember this thought of the sympathetic state (fight or flight) and doing what you can to move back into the parasympathetic state (rest and digest) whenever appropriately possible.

Breathing, Posture and the Nervous System

Breathing and your posture has a profound effect on how the body functions and how much oxygen you take in.

Breathing

Breathing of course allows sufficient amounts of oxygen into the system and when we breathe properly, through what is known as abdominal breathing, we maximise this intake and help to revitalise our cells.

The diaphragm is actually controlled by a nerve at C3, C4 and C5 (which is known as the phrenic nerve) and begins in the neck. 'C' stands for 'Cervical'. This means that when we have a problem with the neck it can indeed affect our breathing.

If our breathing is affected and we are not breathing properly, the amount of carbon dioxide will increase in the body. When this happens the heart rate and blood pressure increases too. When prolonged this can cause the heart to weaken due to it being over worked.

Lack of oxygen can reduce concentration, affect mood and memory and over time motor skills can be affected too. Furthermore, endurance and coordination can be reduced and muscle weakness can become apparent.

In severe cases cell death can occur and then of course death of the whole body.

Breathing properly really is a fundamental part of sustaining good health. Always try to remember to do deep abdominal breathing as this is the proper and natural way to breathe. If you look at a baby you will see that this is how they naturally breathe. You will see the stomach come out first when they take a breath. This is abdominal breathing. This allows the lungs to fill to its full capacity and the maximum amount of oxygen can enter the system. It then is also important to fully empty the lungs after each breath in to allow all of the carbon dioxide out and not funnel it back through the body again.

There is a whole deep science from ancient India known as 'Pranayama' which talks in great detail about the art of breathing correctly. I would highly recommend you look into that and maybe put some of it into use. It really is a solid and effective understanding of the body, breath, energies and how they are all intertwined and affected by just minor adjustments and focus.

Posture

Posture is very important in nerve function because, if we recall, the main 'control room' for the CNS (Central Nervous System) which is the ultimate leader of the body, is housed in the skull and spine.

While poor posture can affect neck, back, joints, spine, muscle load and more, which taxes energy and wears out the body, the nerve implications can be much more important.

When the spine loses its natural curve, our spinal cord becomes stretched which leads to a decrease in blood supply and reduced energy production from the neurones and if continued can deteriorate the communication between the nervous system and the rest of the body.

This of course can be detrimental to health all round.

The importance of this alignment has been echoed for thousands of years in the art of 'Yoga'. Just to briefly mention, Yoga is not about physical exercises or stretching. That is actually just a small part of it. Yoga means 'Union'. This means that in your experience and reality you have become united with all that is.

As I mentioned, Paramahansa Yogananda said that *"The spine and the brain are the altars of God"*.

Paramahansa Yogananda is a yogi, a yoga master. When getting into a meditative state, it is important to keep the back, neck and head in a straight line to allow the proper flow of energy up through the spine into the head.

You can clearly see here that the importance of the spine and what it contains has been known for thousands of years.

Chemicals and the Nervous System

Next, we come to the effect of a wide range of synthetic chemicals on the functioning of the nervous system.

It is a well-established fact that some chemicals have detrimental effects on the functioning, signalling, communication and lifespan of the neurones (the nerve cells).

You will notice that as you read through this book, we refer back to the removal of these toxic chemicals in the solutions we provide. This is because, as we have talked about above, these chemicals move the body into a chemically stressed state and cause a lot of damage.

It is safe to say that synthetic chemicals found in most processed and junk foods, sprayed on our foods, in our water systems, now in the air around us, the products we use for home and body - literally everywhere - is affecting the flow and connectivity of our nerve cells and thus how the complete nervous system works.

Some of the most toxic and dangerous for the nervous system are called 'Neurotoxins'. Neurotoxins are chemicals that specifically affect and poison the neurones. They do this by excessively stimulating them and altering and blocking their correct functioning. In many cases, these chemicals stimulate the neurones to the point of death.

Some of the most dangerous neurotoxins that are

around us in everyday life to be aware of are things like:

- Fluoride (which is found in many toothpastes, mouthwashes and water supplies and has detrimental effects on the endocrine system too)

- Pesticides, Herbicides and Fungicides (sprayed on literally all of our foods - so always soak your fruits and vegetables in water and vinegar - 1 part vinegar to 9 parts water for about 30 minutes to help dissolve some of these residues)

- MSG - Monosodium Glutamate – (found in a wide range of processed foods. As a note, anything that says 'Flavouring' but does not define what exactly that is or means could very much be MSG)

- Aspartame, Sucralose and others (which are artificial sweeteners found in many packaged foods and drinks. You can also get them as standalone sweeteners too - read ALL of your food labels - especially those things that say 'diet' and 'sugar free')

- Aluminium (classed as a heavy metal which can be found in vaccines, drinking water and medications)

- Mercury (which can be found in water, fish products, vaccines and tooth fillings).

With regards to medications, you must be careful

because not only are you bringing a range of foreign, synthetic chemicals into the body, but if you are on many medications, we have no idea how they affect each other and how they react when used together for long periods. There simply has been no long term studies to these affects.

For this reason, taking multiple medications can be a great cause for concern and so should be eradicated where possible with the assistance of a healthcare professional.

If you want to have a healthy and fully functional nervous system, it is of paramount importance that you get these chemicals out of your system and avoid bringing more of them in.

The Gut-Brain Connection

The gut and the brain are very intimately related to one another. If one is damaged, the other too will experience damage.

Let us explore this a little more.

The 'Vagus Nerve' is a very important nerve that starts in the brain and literally connects all of the organs and parts of the body together.

The brain stem, sinuses, voice box, heart, lungs, diaphragm, spleen, liver, stomach, pancreas, kidneys, small and large intestines are all connected via this nerve.

It then connects to other nerves that carry on through the arms and legs.

As it is connected to all these places, it acts like a controller that gives stimulus to all of these parts and then returns information back to the brain for processing.

As you can probably imagine and grasp from what we have said above, this vagus nerve also connects the gut to the brain.

Now, above we laid out the nervous system, but we didn't mention the separate nervous system that is located in the gut. This is known as the 'Enteric Nervous System (ENS)' and it is just as complex and important as the rest of the nervous system.

It is literally like another brain in your gut.

This nervous system is connected to the CNS by the vagus nerve and relays stimulation and information backwards and forwards using this pathway but mainly from the gut up to the brain.

Why is this important?

This is important because if something happens in the gut, such as damage, infection, altered gut biome or other such things, the vagus nerve will react to this and send signals back up to the rest of the nervous system.

This means that if you damage the gut, the vagus nerve in that area can too become damaged and this can lead to damage and lack of sufficient signalling elsewhere in the body and brain as the vagus nerve is connected to all of these parts.

The majority of our body's Serotonin (the feel good chemical) is actually produced in the gut. There is also a close relationship between the gut and conditions such as anxiety and depression because of this.

It is interesting to point out that most children with Autism actually have chronic gut problems too.

It is safe to say that the gut has a profound effect on everything that happens in our body, which is why a lot of focus has been given to the gut in this book and a full plan to help heal the gut has been laid out in the 'Leaky Gut' section.

There are entire books written just about this subject alone, but the essential point I want to get across here is that the gut is very closely linked to the brain and thus it is extremely important to address with regards to physical conditions, neurological conditions and general health and well-being.

Promoting a Healthy Nervous System

Now we have considered the above points, what else can we do to promote a healthy and fully functioning nervous system?

There are a few core things we can do which we have listed below.

- Ensuring the nervous system is clear of strain and interference (which is essentially what we have been talking about above). This should be the first thing that we consider.

- With regards to the vagus nerve we just talked about, to stimulate this and help to ensure it is functioning fully and connected, it is a great idea to hum loudly and to get into chanting. This again, like with meditation, is something that the ancient civilisations knew about and did. They did this to let that resonant frequency vibrate through the entire body and thus it stimulated the vagus nerve from top to bottom.

  One of the best things to do is chant 'AUM'. You open your mouth wide and say 'AHH' like you do when you go to a dentist and they look in your mouth but in a lower pitch so that you can feel it resonating in your lower abdomen around your belly button. Then you simply close your mouth slowly until it is completely closed while still letting the 'AHH' sound out until you run out of breath. You will notice that the sound changes and that the resonance moves from the stomach, to the chest (when the mouth is half closed) and then finally up to the throat (when the mouth is closed).

  This really is a perfect way to stimulate and strengthen that gut-brain connection and thus the connection across the entire nervous system.

- Regular exercise helps to decrease the activity

of the sympathetic nervous system and increase the activity of the parasympathetic nervous system in the long run by increasing communication between the Central and Peripheral Nervous System amongst other things.

- Proper nutrition will help to give the nerve cells what they need to build, repair and stay strong and healthy. To do this they need good fats (which can be found in fish oils, algae oils, avocados, olives, coconut, walnuts, flax seeds, chia seeds and hemp seeds) protein (nuts, seeds, beans, grains), water (preferably fresh and filtered where possible) and the vitamins and minerals we mentioned in the 'Body Essentials' section.

> Saturated fat is important to the nervous system and all the cells of the body. Coconut oil can more than meet your needs for this as most of it is saturated fat and it has a wide range of additional benefits for the entire body.

Omega-3 fatty acids are also very important for the functioning of our system. These can be found predominantly in fish and fish oils in regards to having it in the form that is easy for the body to utilise. It starts in the form of APA but then needs to be converted to EPA and DHA for the body to make use of it. Another non animal based version that has a very good conversion rate also is algae and algae oils, which we talked about a little more in the 'Body Essentials' section.

There are a few things that I would like to give specific mention to, such as:

Selenium is an essential trace mineral that is extremely important for proper functioning and health of your nervous system. It is a trace mineral that helps with the secretion of a range of essential enzymes in the body. One of these substances is 'Glutathione' which is literally the most important antioxidant in the body. It is a very powerful enzyme that protects the cells and neurones from oxidative stress and free radicals.

A free radical happens when an electron becomes singular in the body (normally it is paired) and because of this it can cause damage to other cells and tissues in a chain reaction type style. Glutathione can literally clean this up and stop it from bumping out other molecules in other cells. When used in conjunction with Vitamin E, it is an even more powerful and effective way to keep the cells healthy and vibrant.

Selenium can be obtained from foods such as brazil nuts, seeds, mushrooms, brown rice and oats and you can also get supplemental forms of it. It should definitely be added into your nervous system building regime and should be included in all neurological disorders as part of the treatment.

Given the proper nutrients and environment that contains the nerves, they can indeed regenerate and rebuild themselves.

- Sufficient rest is needed as the body heals and regenerates during deep rest and sleep

- Meditation is also a great way to align the nervous system, put the body into a deep state of rest and out of a stressed state. It also helps the body to release a range of good chemicals and, as we mentioned, the great yogis of India have always said meditation is important and they know that the spine and brain are the most important parts of the system too

Meditation and chanting is really something you should look into for sure. This along with proper nutrition really will help to boost the nervous system.

Thoughts and the Nervous System

The nervous system communicates through trillions upon trillions of electrical and chemical signals. Your thoughts and perceptions alter the electrical and chemical communication in your body. It really is that simple.

If you have ever been scared of something, loved something, excited by something, enjoyed a piece of music or not liked someone, all of these are based on your perception of the world and things around you. Because we have perceptions, ideas and thoughts about our environment and ourselves, these create different pathways of connections within the system that then play out.

Because of this, we can actually make ourselves sick or healthy just with the power of our thoughts. Again, this is something the ancient cultures knew very well, which is why one of the Buddha's first teachings was *'The mind precedes all things'*. Meaning that thought creates our personal reality.

By harbouring negative and destructive thoughts towards ourselves and other people around us, we create connections within our nervous system and body that turns on the stressed state and can keep it there if we do not change our thought patterns.

Similarly, we can heal ourselves and make ourselves feel happy all the time by changing our perceptions about ourselves and the things around us. It is why you can find very happy people who have not a penny to their name, and why you can find very stressed out and unhappy people who have all that they want and need.

It is all about how we manage our internal world.

The Buddha also said this: *'Holding on to anger is like grasping a hot coal with the intent of throwing it at someone else; you are the one who gets burned'* - Again, showing that these kinds of self-created states do us more harm than the person we are sending that negative energy too.

Meditation and detachment should be practiced in order to free yourself of these negative and destructive clutches.

When I say detachment, it does not mean that you do not care about anything around you or have to go and sit in a cave. It simply means that you do not let external factors control you and how you react to situations. You allow yourself to be happy and contented with everything that comes your way whilst you continue to move towards whatever it is that you want out of life.

Worrying and getting stressed about things only hinders your performance and ability to deal with situations.

It does not help anything.

Your thought patterns really are so important in how your nervous system communicates and how the body reacts so be sure to do what you can to move into a positive, happy and contented state of mind. This really is paramount for deep healing to occur.

Holistic Immune System Building

Three core principles
When healing the body, there are always three things that should be remembered and considered. These are:

- **Cleansing**
- **Fortifying and**
- **Preserving**

Cleansing comprises of removing all of the toxic, obstructive and non-productive things that may be present in the tissues, blood, cells and organs of the body.

Fortifying comprises of repopulating the body with what it needs that might have been lost over the duration of the illness or condition. This can be in the form of vitamins, minerals, good bacteria, fluids and other such things.

Preserving is all about sustaining the re-established healthy environment in and around the body that contributes to a long and healthy life.

Throughout this book we shall be essentially addressing these three core principles.

Remembering and utilising these three core principles is what is at the heart of all natural healthcare approaches.

Layout of the Immune System

The immune system is a whole network of specialised cells and organs spread across the body that are designed to detect, protect against and eradicate invaders of all types and heal any damage that occurs.

A great way to look at the immune system is like the front line of defence and the military system of the body.

As I said, the immune system is spread across the entire body. It is important to note though that 80% of that is located in the gut in the small intestines. You then have immune cells in all of the tissues of the body, circulating in the blood and then you also have the drainage system that helps to clean out all of the rubbish and toxins named the lymphatic system. We will talk more about the lymphatic system in a minute.

The immune system can be categorised into two main parts. Let's have a quick look at the two:

- The 'Innate' Immune System and

- The 'Adaptive' or 'Acquired' Immune System

Innate

The Innate immune system is the first line of defence. This is a generalised set of immune cells that recognise when an intruder first comes into the body. It recognises general groups of pathogens (invaders) such as viruses, bacteria and parasites and then mounts the initial attack. It then signals for the other immune cells to come and help with the invasion.

Adaptive

This second system is known as the Adaptive Immune System. It is named this because it contains cells that recognise pathogens and problems from the past and can create specific responses that will fight that specific attack. When it comes into contact with something new, it will remember this the next time it comes along.

These two systems work in partnership to keep you healthy and invasion free as much as it can.

The Lymphatic System

Finally, we have the 'Lymphatic System'. The lymphatic system takes all of the toxins and rubbish from the tissues and puts it into the blood stream where it can be disposed of. It is comprised of a range of organs, such as the tonsils, thymus gland, spleen, vessels and ducts. The vessels spread across the body like the circulatory system and cover the main body area, legs, arms and neck.

The lymphatic system needs movement in order to be stimulated and work properly. This is another reason why exercise and even light things like walking are very beneficial. Deep breathing is also another thing that stimulates its movement.

Moving through the GI Tract

We need to talk about foods that are going to help boost the immune system in a natural way but before we do that we have to ensure that the foods you consume are going to be able to be utilised by the body and thus used to strengthen the immunity.

Otherwise, if the body cannot absorb the nutrition, it could all be futile.

Firstly, we have to ensure we have a healthy and adequate amount of stomach acid (hydrochloric acid) and a healthy GI tract (intestines).

For a healthy amount of stomach acid to be produced we must ensure we have adequate amounts of Vitamin B1 (Thiamine), Zinc, Iodine, Salt and Body Electricity. For more on these and how to get enough into your system, please see the 'Acid Reflux' section of this book.

Next, we need to ensure that once the food has been broken down in the stomach properly, the nutrients can be absorbed by the small intestines and transferred into the body for use by the cells and tissues.

To ensure you have a healthy and strong intestinal tract please see the 'Leaky Gut' section of the book where we have gone into healing the gut in much more detail.

Once we have ensured that the food is being broken down properly and that the small intestines are absorbing the nutrients efficiently, we then of course want to ensure the nutrients being absorbed are of the highest quality. So for this we want to consume organic, fresh and predominantly raw fruits, vegetables, nuts, seeds and good fats wherever possible.

This is the winning combination.

These categories of foods in the right combination will cleanse, fortify and preserve the body, hitting all three of our core principles of Cleansing, Fortifying and Preserving.

Throughout the book you will see me repeating this, so when you see this remember that more vegetables over fruits is always a good idea, especially the consumption of dark leafy green vegetables.

So, why are these foods the 'winning combination'? Let us talk about each of these categories of food.

Firstly we have the organic and raw vegetables
The reason we recommend that you eat predominantly raw and organic vegetables is because when you eat foods raw you take in their full amount of available enzymes, vitamins, minerals and fibre that are very beneficial to the body. When we cook food we actually break down these enzymes and reduce the amount of vitamins and minerals available and so are not getting the full healing potential from the foods we eat.

This is the same situation with fruits too. The more you can eat fruits and vegetables raw, the better the healing and vitalising effects on the body.

It can be harder to digest raw food and so for this reason it is advisable to blend where ever possible. Juicing is very good too, but when we juice we take out all of the fibre which is actually very good for our gut and helps to keep the colon clean.

So if you have trouble eating the raw foods, blend them up together and drink them. You can actually manage to consume more this way too.

We then recommend organic because organically grown food has an increased amount of vitamins and minerals in the foods when compared to their conventionally grown counterparts. This has to do with the living ecosystems of bacteria's that are present in organic soil and the higher levels of minerals present.

Organic farmers culture the soil in a way that allows the good bacteria to grow and thrive there. Whereas conventional farmers use lots of synthetic fertilisers and pesticides and other such things that partly destroys this ecosystem, if not completely, but can increase yields of the plant which is why they do it.

While organic farmers do still use pesticides in many cases, it is generally in less amounts and not as harmful a chemical as what is used in conventional farming.

For these reasons we always recommend that you eat raw and organic wherever possible.

Next, we have the seeds and nuts
These foods are part of the winning combination because seeds contain high amounts of vitamins, minerals and protein that the body needs in order to be strong and healthy, internally and externally.

Another way to get a lot more out of the seeds we eat is to 'sprout' them.

This is a process where we allow the seeds to just about start growing which activates a whole lot more of the nutrients in the seed and plant.

Other benefits that come with sprouting your seeds are things like making them easier to digest and making it easier to assimilate the increased available enzymes and nutrients in the seed.

You can try by getting started with seeds such as sunflower and pumpkin and seeing what you think.

Finally, we have the 'good fats'
A lot of this has been covered in the'Body Essentials' section, but we shall just briefly mention it again.

The body needs fats in order to build healthy and fully functioning cells, and this includes saturated fats too. They are generally used to create the membrane of the cells (the outer layer) and help to conduct the flow of information in and out of the cell.

Whilst we may have heard that saturated fats are 'bad' fats, this is not necessarily true. The problem with saturated fat is when we have too much of it. For example, when you eat lots of fatty meats, like sausages, bacon and the sort, this can lead to having too much saturated fat which is also mixed with animal protein and this becomes very acidic in the system, which is why we are talking about the 'good' fats.

The healthiest source of saturated fat, and one that is more than sufficient for what the cells in your body need, is coconut oil. Coconut oil is around 80 – 90%

saturated fat but comes with a vast range of internal and external healing benefits which are well documented now.

Fats we want to avoid are those that have been modified in some way. These are the trans fats and hydrogenated oils that are predominantly found in your processed and junk foods.

As well as a good source of saturated fats, we also want to consume a good amount of omega 3 fatty acids too.

The best sources are krill oil, fish oils, algae oils, ground chia and flax seeds and wakame seaweed.

Ok, so now we know about the winning combinations of foods. Let's address a few more specific foods that will help in building your immune system

The best foods and substances to build the immune system are things such as berries which are high in antioxidants and anthocyanins.

Anthocyanins are a type of flavonoid (which we will get to in a minute) and is responsible for the red-blue pigment that gives berries and other fruits their colour - the darker the fruit, the more that is present and the better the effects – for example blueberries over strawberries. Anthocyanins are very good in protecting the body from disease and strengthening the immune system.

In plants they are used to protect it from UV radiation.

Other foods include garlic and onions and their active ingredient 'Allicin' which is a sulphur containing compound that is responsible for their infection, fungal, bad bacteria and parasitic fighting capabilities which takes the strain off of your immune cells so they can better protect the body from new incoming problems.

Mushrooms are very interesting. Mushrooms are a type of fungus and are actually a bridge between us and the plant world and so are actually closer to us in terms of evolution than plants.

They contain a whole host of immune building and fungal, bacterial, viral, parasitic and even yeast killing compounds. Mushrooms can actually get the same bacteria's and viruses as we can and so they have developed a sophisticated and very strong defence against these things that are then very beneficial to us too. Did you know that the antibiotic penicillin actually comes from fungi?

Fungi are nature's cleaners, they help to break down decaying organic compounds and turn them back to soil.

If it wasn't for fungi we would be swimming up to our eye balls in dead organic matter. Mushrooms also have the same effect in your body, they help to break down and clear out damaged tissue and also harmful microbes, bacteria's and viruses. They also facilitate the rebuilding of cells and nerves and so are extremely beneficial for the system and increase the response of and number of the white bloods cells (the immune cells) in the body.

Mushrooms protect the organs, improve blood flow and heart health, help to normalise blood sugar levels, improve and help heal the respiratory organs and so much more.

Essentially, you want to be eating a good amount of mushrooms all the time. Try mixing and matching different mushrooms too to reap the increased benefits of bringing different ones together. Some of the best ones are Shiitake, Chaga, Lion's Mane and Reishi mushroom.

Turmeric is an important spice that you definitely want to add to your immune boosting arsenal.

Turmeric has an active ingredient called 'Curcumin' which has powerful anti-inflammatory, anti-viral, anti-bacterial and anti-parasitic effects. It helps with the activation, deployment and effectiveness of all the immune cells (which is why it helps against parasites and bacteria) and helps with the functioning and health of the body's organs.

This really is a super spice that will boost your immune system and keep you strong and healthy. It can also be used topically for infections and other external problems and has proven to be very useful against cancer.

Resveratrol is a compound that is actually produced by certain plants to help them fight off injury, infections and the harmful effects of continuous UV exposure.

This compound can be found in grapes predominantly, more in red grapes, and can help to regulate the production and deployment of immune cells and therefor helps to keep the body functioning at its best whilst keeping the skin and organs vibrant and healthy (which makes sense when we look at the reason the compound is in the plants).

This is the reason that people say one glass of wine a day is good for you. It is not that the alcoholic wine itself is good for you, but that wine is made from grapes that contain the resveratrol and you get a concentrated amount in the wine. Alcohol in general is not good for the body and so it is better to go directly to the source and just eat the organic and fresh red grapes.

Other foods high in resveratrol are peanuts, blueberries, cranberries and raw cocoa.

Flavonoids are compounds found in plants that help the plant with cell communication and act as antioxidants for them and therefor are great for detoxifying the body and are also anti-inflammatory.

Flavonoids are quite a wide range of phytonutrients, which essentially are there to protect and help the plant stay healthy and infection free. They fall into subcategories too, but we won't go into them here.

Instead, we will just list a range of foods that these protective compounds can be found in, and these are:

Onions, apples, garbanzo beans, almonds, sweet potatoes, grain quinoa, bananas, most berries, peaches, pears, parsley, bell peppers, celery, oranges, grapefruit, lemons, cabbage, plums, raw cocoa, kidney beans, spinach and kale.

Selenium is an essential trace mineral that is extremely important in literally all functions of the body, from protection to enzyme creation.

With regards to the immune system it is important for all functions of it. It is the trace mineral that allows and stimulates new immune cells to start proliferating so that they can protect the body.

Selenium works to protect the nucleus of all cells as well and transports amino acids into the cell for use. It is literally the first line of protection and primary heavy metal and toxin detoxifier for the cells too.

It is also a very important mineral for the healthy functioning of the eyes, liver, brain, thyroid and heart amongst others.

You can consume selenium in conjunction with the amino acid methionine (found in quinoa, spirulina and sesame seeds) as this will further increase the production of 'Glutathione' as both act as precursors to it. Glutathione is the body's most powerful antioxidant.s

A Good Night's Sleep
A good night's sleep is one of the most important

things that your body needs in order to be and stay healthy.

A good night's sleep will allow healing and repair to take place and this is because when you are sleeping, your body relaxes fully and thus tensions and strains that are generally on the body during the day are drastically reduced, especially those caused by emotional stresses.

This then will also allow the body to recharge and the immune system to work at its best.

Finally, I would just like to refer you back to the list of foods we gave at the end of 'The Body Essentials' section of the book. As well as taking into account the above information, do not forget to do your best to add these into your diet as well to ensure your body is getting what it needs.

Ok, so now we have addressed those important subjects it is now time to get into the main part of this book, and that is addressing these conditions that many of us are seeing in our lives, our families lives and all over the world.

So let's jump straight in with the most common diseases and conditions from A-Z.

Acid Reflux

What is it?

Acid reflux is a condition where the acid that is in the stomach (hydrochloric acid) is able to move upward into the Oesophagus (the pipe leading from the mouth to the stomach) and because this pipe is not coated with a protective mucus layer in the same way the stomach is, the acid burns the oesophagus which causes the 'heart burn' feeling that is associated with it.

When persistent, the oesophagus can also become inflamed causing a continuous heart burn like feeling when eating due to the irritation.

So, what causes it?

Contrary to belief, Acid Reflux is not generally caused by too much acid in the stomach.

Instead it is actually due to the stomach acid not being strong enough or not enough present in many cases. A lack of sufficient stomach acid can also be called 'Hypochlorhydria' which produces the same symptoms as what we know to be Acid Reflux.

Let me explain in a little more detail:

At the bottom of the stomach, at the antrum, is a kind of sensor that senses the pH of the acid in the stomach. When there is a strong level of stomach acid between 2.5pH - 3.0pH or lower (more acidic) the sphincter between the stomach and oesophagus is then signalled to shut to stop the acid rising up into the oesophagus and burning it.

There can be other causes for this sphincter between the oesophagus and stomach not to close, which include obesity, sometimes pregnancy and bacterial infection and growth in the area (which can come from infections and bacterial overgrowth in the mouth too), but generally it is the reason we mentioned above.

So, what can cause the decrease in acidity of our stomach acid?

Generally it is because of a deficiency in one of the 5 things that are needed for the cells in the stomach to produce sufficient hydrochloric acid, these are Vitamin B1 (Thiamine), Iodine, Zinc, Salt (Sodium and Chloride) and the body's natural electricity. When any of these become low or you become deficient in these, the problem can then occur.

So pharmaceutical medication to suppress the acid is generally not the answer here.

Medications such as 'antacids', which are regularly prescribed when people go to the doctor complaining of ongoing heart burn or acid reflux, reduce the amount of hydrochloric acid produced and are actually worsening the condition and not addressing the real cause of the problem. In many cases these drugs are actually bringing on a host of other problems too.

Reasons to not reduce the stomachs acid is because hydrochloric acid plays a very important role for the body. It sterilises food coming in to the body from any harmful bacterias, it helps to start the breakdown of the food into its individual amino acids, vitamins and minerals and helps to convert the enzymes needed in the stomach and GI Tract (intestines).

If you have poor acid in the stomach, proteins cannot be broken down into their individual amino acids and therefore cannot be absorbed properly by the body as the body can only absorb amino acids.

It is also important to point out here that stomach acid generally decreases with age, not increases, so when we hear of older people complaining of this condition more and more, we must look at their nutrient intake and levels.

Symptoms

All of these following symptoms may not be felt all at once, but those with acid reflux can experience some of these symptoms:

'Heartburn' which is a burning or acidic sensation that is felt in the chest and sometimes up into the throat, chest pain, difficulty swallowing, sore throat, food or liquid coming back up a little in the throat and a lump like feeling in the throat.

Solutions

Address it from the core cause. Ensure there is no deficiency in Vitamin B1 (Thiamine), Iodine, Zinc, Salt and Electricity in the body.

'Vitamin B1' can be found in Flax Seeds, Sunflower

Seeds, Brown Rice, Asparagus, Kale, Cauliflower and Beans.

'Iodine' can be found in Seafood, Kelp and most Seaweeds, Cranberries, Navy Beans and Potatoes.

'Zinc' can be found in Seafood, Spinach, Pumpkin Seeds, Squash Seeds, Nuts, Raw Cocoa Powder, Mung Beans and Mushrooms.

'Salt' which should only be in limited, small amounts is best to be obtained from Sea Salt, not table salt.

'Electricity' - when we say electricity we are looking at what stimulates the best flow of the body's natural electricity, which is greatly assisted by alkaline and organic plant based foods, which is why it is best to eat good amounts of fresh, organic and raw fruits and vegetables to get the highest amount of energy from them and help the body maintain its slightly alkaline state which increases the electrical output.

Eating organic fruits, vegetables, nuts, seeds and good fats will also give you all of the nutrients you need to reduce any deficiencies. Highly acidic and mucus forming foods may make things worse so avoid processed and junk foods, fatty and cheap meats, lots of dairy and high intake of sugar and foods that turn to sugar such as wheat (and foods made with wheat), white rice, white potatoes and other starchy foods.

We also know that when the blood is in an acidic state, the body has less electricity and is much more prone to disease than when in an optimal slightly alkaline state (7.4pH).

Remember when eating meals to not drink anything around 10 minutes before the meal and 30 minutes after. This is to ensure we do not dilute the stomach acid further.

Once we have addressed these, we then want to do what we can to stop taking antacids and other medications that reduce the acidity of the stomach for the reasons mentioned above. Remember to do this with the supervision of a healthcare professional.

With those in check, we can then ensure to keep dental hygiene up to a good standard to avoid infection and gum diseases which can then affect the sphincter between the oesophagus and the stomach, not to mention the rest of the gut too.

See the 'Gum Disease' section for more info on that and dental hygiene.

Just to be thorough, I should also mention that it may be a good idea to look at the gut to ensure that the nutrients you are taking in through food are actually being absorbed into the body. You can get tests at your doctors to check for any problems with the gut.

If it turns out that you do have some issues with the gut, please read our 'Leaky Gut' section of this book that explains in detail how to go about healing and repairing this area.

By following these steps you should notice a marked difference in the condition of Acid Reflux.

Alzheimer's Disease

What is it?
Alzheimer's disease is a neurological condition in which 'amyloid plaques' and 'neurofibrillary tangles' form in the brain that interrupt and destroy neurones which then lead to the issues associated with this condition (mentioned in the symptoms below).

What does this really mean?

In simple terms it means that neurones (the nerve cells) are getting tangled up and dying off in large amounts and that plaques (clusters of small bits of proteins) build up in-between the nerve cells and continue the deterioration and tangling/destruction of the neurones.

Ideally, not something you want happening.

So, what causes it?
One of the causes that lead up to the condition of Alzheimer's is exposure to toxic chemicals, known as neurotoxins, and to heavy metal exposure.

When these things get into the system, they affect the signalling, communication and functioning of the neurones and in many cases overstimulate the neurones to the point of death. Thus, this leads to the malfunctioning, deterioration and continuing death of the cells and also extensive nerve damage.

The current leading thought in the medical field is that there is a malfunctioning or abnormally processed protein called 'tau' that is involved with sending information from the neurone body down the axon.

It would make sense then that something that overstimulates and makes these neurones act uncontrollably would have an effect on these processes.

This is exactly what neurotoxins do. Which is why they have the name. 'Neuro' means relating to the nervous system and 'toxin' stands for poison. So a neurotoxin is essentially a nervous system poison.

Some of the most dangerous neurotoxins to be aware of are things like:

- Fluoride (which is found in many toothpastes, mouthwashes and water supplies)

- Pesticides (sprayed on our foods)

- Herbicides and Fungicides (also sprayed on our foods)

- MSG (Monosodium Glutamate - found in a wide range of foods - as a note, anything that says 'Flavouring' in the ingredients list but is not defined as what that is could very much be MSG)

- Aspartame and Sucralose (which are artificial sweeteners found in many foods and drinks - read ALL of your food labels - especially those things that say 'diet' and 'sugar free')

- Aluminium (found in vaccines, drinking water

and medications)

- Mercury (which can be found in water, fish products, vaccines and tooth fillings).

It is very common to find a build-up of aluminium in the brains of those who suffer from Alzheimer's disease.

After looking at this list it is not hard to see why we are witnessing an epidemic in this condition. These chemicals are literally everywhere and in most of the things we consume and use in today's world.

Essentially it is best to avoid processed foods, medications where possible, vaccines, toxic and synthetic chemicals and other such things of this nature. This should be the first step and concern for those with Alzheimer's.

Another cause that has been linked to this condition is chronic elevated blood sugar. This is because when there is a rise in blood sugar, neurone firing in the brain is also increased. Under normal conditions this is ok, but when there is a sudden rise in blood sugar they fire too much which increases the 'beta-amyloid' protein (the protein that leads to the plaques in the brain) and thus increases the chances of these tangles occurring.

This means that people with chronic high blood sugar and of course diabetes have a greater chance of developing Alzheimer's, which is something that is known today.

Symptoms

Symptoms can include memory loss, loss of ability to problem solve, confusion, trouble comprehending things that used to be easy, difficulty completing tasks, issues with speaking and writing, poor judgement, misplacing items, withdrawal from activities and other people, forgetting people and things and changes in mood and personality.

Of course, all of these symptoms may not be present at once, but these are the potential symptoms that can develop.

Solutions

The first and foremost thing that must be considered when looking at a solution to Alzheimer's disease is to reduce the toxicity that the person is subjected to and detox the already accumulated toxic chemicals.

Detox

This means firstly addressing the foods and drinks that come in to the body that contain chemicals. This would be things like literally all processed foods, junk foods, inorganic foods, fizzy drinks, unfiltered water, artificial sweeteners/colours and preservatives and other foods and drinks with chemicals in them.

With these eliminated, we then want to reduce the external toxins we are exposed to which can be present in:

- Toiletries such as toothpastes, washing products, creams and deodorants, all of which have natural alternatives

- Household washing products that use synthetic chemicals, which includes for clothes, dishes and cutlery, carpets, sofas, bed and windows as these chemicals will then stay present in your home. Again these all have natural alternatives

- Outdoor pollution. While this may be a hard thing to avoid, it is important to try and reduce the amount of pollution you breathe into the system. While it may not be fashionable, it may be beneficial to wear air pollution masks if you live or work in highly polluted areas

- Unfiltered tap water. Whilst clean of bacteria and viruses, tap water has been found to have traces of heavy metals such as aluminium present in it and so you should also filter the water that you drink. You can use something like a 'Reverse Osmosis Filter' for this

- Vaccinations which contain a whole host of toxic chemicals including aluminium

- Medications

If you are on medications, do your best to reduce or completely remove these from the system as these contain chemicals which will slow down the rate of any recovery and repair. Remember if you are going to attempt to come off of medications, you should always do this with the supervision of a professional healthcare provider.

Never just go 'cold turkey' and just stop taking your

medications as this can lead to a range of adverse and potentially dangerous side effects.

With these factors considered and eradicated from entering the system, we then want to focus on detoxing the already accumulated toxins.

You can help to detox the body and keep the cells and neurones healthy with fresh, organic and preferably raw fruits and vegetables, especially dark leafy greens and foods high in antioxidants such as berries, grapes, raw cocoa, carrots, oranges and squash plus other foods high in Vitamin C and E (doing juices and blends are a great way to get these into your system quickly and much more easily as energy will not be spent on digesting them to release their nutrients).

It is important to take things such as garlic, turmeric, onions, omega-3's (found in good amounts in fish oil, krill oil, algae oils and ground chia and flax seeds), Vitamin D and Vitamin B12 which again will help the cells stay clean, healthy and strong.

The best source of Vitamin D is of course the sun.

Remember our 'winning combination' of foods from the 'Holistic Immune System Building' section of this book?

Utilise this as much as you can.

As a side note, it is a good idea to wash your fruit and vegetables in water with some vinegar to help disintegrate some of the pesticide residues left on them. It is good to do about a 9:1 ratio, with 9 being water, 1 being vinegar.

Another important factor to add in here is the use of Selenium which can be obtained from foods but also higher amounts in supplements. Selenium acts as a precursor to a very powerful antioxidant that will help to repair some of the damage to the nerves and detox the accumulation of heavy metals and toxins.

As Alzheimer's has also been classed as a kind of 'Diabetes of the Brain' by some professionals, it has been shown that because there is a lack of insulin getting into the brain to help with energy assimilation, the cells can actually get there energy from 'ketones' which are released when 'medium chained triglycerides' are metabolised in the liver. Ketones are like an energy source that is used when fat is metabolised for energy instead of glucose. This can be found in our favourite saturated fat, coconut oil.

This should be added to the new diet and always consumed in its pure form though, not altered or hydrogenated.

Finally in this detoxing stage, you want to keep the body moving to stimulate the lymphatic system as it needs movement in order for it to work and do its job of removing waste materials from the tissues of the body. For this reason, light exercise is also beneficial. Even if it is just walking a little each day, it is important to do what you can, but do not overdo it or strain yourself.

Keeping the mind active
With toxin exposure drastically reduced and nutritional

and detoxifying foods now in the diet, we now want to ensure to keep the mind active with mental exercises such as puzzle games, problem solving tasks, even working towards worthwhile goals and other things to keep the mind active and in use. There are even brain training games which can be downloaded as apps.

The mind is an amazing tool and, if you put it to work for you, can yield astonishing results. Neurones rebuild, new pathways can be established and new things and ways of thinking can always be learned.

You can train your mind to think in a certain way, which will then affect how your nervous system functions, which in turn will affect how your immune system functions and how communication between cells happen. For these reasons, meditation is a powerful tool to help keep your mind, nervous system and immune system fresh, vitalised and healthy.

You can then take further actions to reduce stress in your life. This can be accomplished through a range of things such as taking walks in fresh air (going through wooded areas and the beach are good places), meditation, yoga, listening to relaxing music and other such things that will reduce your emotional stresses, which if left unchecked, can reduce your body's ability to protect you, clean up any free radical damage and reduce ability to clean up infection and disease, which leads to more stresses on the body. All of this will reduce your ability to heal and thus speed up deterioration and slow down any possible progress that can be made.

If you have any other conditions, it is also beneficial to

reduce the impact of these on the body as they will put further strain and stresses on the immune system, which strives to keep the body healthy and strong.

By putting all of these suggestions into use, the onset and symptoms of Alzheimer's can be reduced over long periods of time. If you are worried about the possibility of developing Alzheimer's disease then these are very powerful preventative measures.

If you can supply the body with the raw materials that it needs to rebuild cells and then give it the right environment in which to do so, diseases of the body can be reverted.

The body has and always will have an innate ability to heal and repair itself so do what you can to facilitate this.

Arthritis (Osteo)

What is it?
Osteoarthritis is the most common type of arthritis and is a condition in which the joints of the body become affected and start to deteriorate.

The cartilage deteriorates and excess bone can grow, called spurs, in the joints. With the deterioration of the cartilage (the smooth coating on the ending of bones in the joints) bones then rub against each other causing inflammation, which leads to further deterioration, stiffness and pain.

This generally happens to the knee joints, spine, hips and hands but can happen in any joint on the body.

This type of arthritis generally happens in one joint at a time and it is not always mirrored (such as both knees or both hips) like it is in Rheumatoid Arthritis (RA) which is classified as an 'Auto-Immune Disease' (see the 'Rheumatoid Arthritis' section for more on that type of arthritis).

So, what causes it?
This condition can be known as the 'wear and tear' condition because it is generally affected by things such as being over-weight (which puts continuous pressure on the joints) and repetitive strain of the joint.

Other causes can include hormonal changes and nutritional deficiencies that can lead to a change in the amount of 'synovial fluid' in the joint (synovial fluid is the fluid that surrounds and feeds the cartilage in the joint).

Bone density also has a role to play here as a reduction in bone density will lead to deterioration and brittle bones. The bone density can become reduced due to a number of things, such as a lack of nutrients in the body, a decrease in stomach acid (see the 'Acid Reflux' section) which will stop the efficient absorption of calcium as the stomach acid is needed for this process and, finally, an acidic diet which will make the blood acidic and thus calcium and other minerals will be leeched out of the bone in order to neutralise the pH of the blood.

All of these things can and will cause deterioration of the bones and joints and lead to osteoarthritis.

Solutions

The solution is based around clearing already accumulated waste from the body, reducing the intake of further toxins, increasing bone density and fortifying the body with the nutrients it needs to rebuild and heal.

So let us address each of these areas in a little more detail.

Clearing accumulated waste

It is important to keep the body moving in order to stimulate the lymphatic system which helps to clear waste out of the body. This process of removing any waste products helps to slow deterioration.

This can be done by rubbing the affected part and keeping the body moving with light exercise such as some walking and some light activity to stimulate cleaning and filtering in that area.

Reducing intake of further toxins
It is very important to adjust the diet in order to help the body do what it does best, and that is to heal. It is advisable to take out junk foods, processed foods, acidic foods, fried foods, high sugar foods, foods filled with chemicals and fatty and cheap meats and certainly GMO foods as all of these will deteriorate the body further and put the body into a chemically stressed state.

When the body is in a stressed state, healing becomes very difficult.

Next be aware of the drinks you consume. It is advisable to move away from artificially sweetened/coloured or preserved drinks, drinks with added sugar, fizzy drinks and caffeinated drinks. Avoiding these things will reduce the body's chemically stressed state and change the internal environment to one that is conducive to healing.

The things you put on your skin (in the form of washing products and deodorants - which there are natural alternatives for), and other things you put into your system (such as chemicals in toothpaste and mouthwash) should also be considered and adapted.

Remember, the aim here is to move away from harmful chemicals that accumulate in the system, move away from anything that makes the blood acidic and move the body out of a stressed state, whether that be chemically, emotionally or physically.

Increasing bone density

To help increase bone density it is important to try your best to move away from pharmaceutical medications as they can deplete and drain nutrients out of the system which will put the body into a chemically stressed state again and thus work against the natural healing capabilities and health of the body.

Boosting nutrition and intake of alkalising foods will help in increasing bone density by moving the pH of the blood away from an acidic state and thus not unnecessarily taking calcium out of the bones.

Some light exercise will be healthy for the body as it gets out toxins but also some kind of resistance training can be good because when the bones have loads on them it increases the bone density but ensure to have good form and not to strain when doing exercises. Try not to do more than you are able and feel comfortable doing no matter how little that may be.

Fortifying the body with nutrients

The things listed here will also help to clear the accumulated toxins in the body too.

The best foods for fortifying the body and increasing bone density will be organic, fresh, unprocessed and preferably raw fruits and vegetables, especially dark leafy greens as these are high in calcium and nutrients that the body needs. These foods will help the body maintain its naturally slightly alkaline state which helps with calcium absorption too instead of taking it from your bones.

Remember to soak fruit and veg in water and vinegar to dissolve as much of the pesticide residue as possible.

Some people think that you can only get calcium from dairy, but this is not true. You can get more than enough calcium from plant based foods, such as beans, dark leafy greens and nuts.

This will also help to replenish the nutrients in the synovial fluid around the cartilage and joint to keep the area healthy.

Finally, drink lots of fresh and filtered water and have a sufficient intake of Omega-3 fatty acids and saturated fats which is another important factor for aiding you with calcium absorption and helping cells rebuild healthily. The most active kind of this can be obtained from krill oil, fish oils and from algae oils and ground chia and flax seeds too and be sure to keep Vitamin D levels up in the body.

These are some of the best ways to rebuild and keep the joints and bones healthy and thus treat osteoarthritis.

Asthma

What is it?

Asthma is a condition in which the person has a hypersensitive airway which can lead the system to overreact to things that others might not react to and because of this breathing can become very difficult.

The airway of the sufferer becomes inflamed and constricted because of the muscles contracting around the airways. There is also an excessive build-up of mucus. All of this leads to a much more difficult time with breathing.

So, what causes it?

There are many triggers for asthma sufferers such as pollen, dust, animal hair, smoke, colds, stress, anxiety and other allergies due to the system being in a hypersensitive state.

So, essentially, because this is an allergy based and hypersensitive state, we want to start by looking at the gut, especially if you have other allergies too, as this can be the cause for many allergy based reactions and cause the hypersensitivity in the first place.

You can get this checked at your local doctors. If it turns out that you do have a problem with the gut, such as inflammation, damage or leakiness, be sure to check out our 'Leaky Gut' section of this book for a detailed and natural way to heal and fortify this area.

Then as this is a hypersensitive state also, the nervous system should then be checked.

Symptoms

Symptoms can include shortness of breath, wheezing, regular coughing, tiredness and weakness after exertion, mood changes, pain or tightness in chest.

Solutions

You may think we would just advise to address the lungs as this is where the problem occurs, but breathing is actually controlled by the nervous system. For this reason, this is where we must start.

We have gone into great detail about how to cleanse, vitalise and preserve the nervous system in our 'Holistic Nervous System Building' section of the book.

Please be sure to read this section and implement the advice given there.

In addition to the above, there are some more things you can do specifically related to asthma, such as:

-   Eliminating mucus building foods such as dairy, fatty, inorganic meats and acidic foods.

This is why we recommend fresh, organic and preferably raw fruits and vegetables, especially an abundance of dark leafy greens, as this will help to clear up the mucus and at the same time nourish the nervous system and gradually help move it out of a hypersensitive state especially as we continue to move the body out of a stressed state.

- Avoid soy and cut down on grains containing gluten like wheat, barley and rye as these can damage the good bacteria in the gut and the gut lining.

- Cut down on sugar and foods that turn to sugar in the system (generally starchy foods) such as foods and drinks with added sugar, white potatoes, white rice, flour and those things made from wheat grains such as breads and pastas.

- Keep your home and places you spend your time clean and dust free where possible to reduce any external pressures on your system. This includes reducing the amount of toxic fumes and pollution you are subjected to if this can at all be helped.

- Reduce stressful situations in your life as stress puts the body into the sympathetic state ('fight or flight') and so does not allow the nervous system and the rest of the body to relax and move away from its hypersensitive state.

You can try and reduce stress through things such as meditation, yoga, going for walks in nature, listening to relaxing music, refocusing your mind on the positive aspects of your life and being around people that bring out the best in you, not the worst.

We want to increase mucus clearing and anti-inflammatory foods such as pumpkin seeds, ginger, onions, garlic, honey, pineapple, grapefruit, substances high in omega 3 fatty acids such as krill oil and algae oil and ground chia and flax seeds and increasing our intake of Vitamins A,C and E + lots of fresh and filtered water (all as raw and organic as possible).

A very powerful anti-oxidant to include in this solution is Selenium. Selenium is used as a precursor to a very important antioxidant used by the body so be sure to get sufficient amounts of this trace mineral. It can be obtained from certain foods or it can be obtained from supplemental form.

Another great thing you can do to help with Asthma is to do deep breathing, called abdominal breathing, to help get good amounts of oxygen into the system. Doing this over a bowl of steaming hot water with a towel over your head and a few drops of tea tree essential oil in the water is another good way to break up mucus, clear away any possible bacterial build up and open up the airways.

As we mentioned in the causes section, as this is allergy based, if after going to your doctor and finding out if you have any issues with your gut, if it turns out that you do indeed have issues there it is advisable to go about cleansing and fortify the GI tract (intestines) to ensure no more allergy causing reactions continue to happen in the body. For full and detailed information on this please see our 'Leaky Gut' section of this book.

If you do your best to implement these steps, you should notice a drastic difference in the condition.

Autism

What is it?

Autism is a neurological developmental condition that affects people from an early age. It is characterised by difficulty in communicating, forming relationships, social interactions and language.

It is included in what is known as the 'Autism Spectrum' as it contains many different conditions that range in severity such as Asperger's, Childhood Disintegrative Disorder and Rett Syndrome.

So, what causes it?

It is important to understand the guts relation in regards to neurological development and disease.

The gut consists of trillions of bacteria, both good and bad, but generally a higher degree of good over bad. If we was to estimate the ratio of bacteria in the body to our own cells, the bacteria would outweigh us at about 10:1.

In the gut a range of neurotransmitters are produced and one of these is serotonin. Whilst serotonin is also produced in the brain, 90-95% of it is actually produced in the gut and is used for the peristalsis wave that helps to push food through the intestines.

As we saw in the 'Holistic Nervous System Building' section, the gut is connected to the brain via the vagus nerve and it is along this pathway that serotonin also travels up to the brain to essentially let it know what is happening in the gut. We also know that serotonin across the body plays an important role in memory, learning, mood, sleep, appetite, digestion and can have effects on the endocrine system and cardiovascular system too.

For this reason it is very important that you have a good production of serotonin in the gut for good brain health.

We also see mirrored affects too such as when the gut is inflamed, the brain too can become inflamed and the person experiences 'brain fog' which again shows this tight relationship between the gut and the brain.

It is important to note the gut and brain connection here because it is found in literally all Autistic children that they have chronic gut problems and a 'leaky gut'.

So now we have established that the gut is of great importance here. What can damage the gut?

As we mentioned, the gut is balanced between good and bad bacteria. In a healthy gut this is leaning on the side of good. So this balance of the trillions of bacteria is very important. We call this ecosystem the gut biome.

There are a range of things that can disturb this biome and cause either damage to the gut lining and thus things that are not supposed to enter the blood stream, now can (called Leaky Gut) or can cause the increase of bad bacteria which will cause problems with chemical production, nutrient absorption and signalling to the brain.

When this happens, as 80% of the immune system is in the gut, immunity is also compromised and put out of balance which reduces its ability to protect the body which can lead to oxidative stress. This essentially means that free radicals are not cleared up enough by antioxidants in the body and thus can cause a lot of damage to tissues and cells. This can and does affects every part of the body, including brain health.

Other factors that can alter the gut biome include:

GMO foods – As you would have read in the GMO part of the 'Understanding The Epidemic' section of the book, the 'rogue' or 'unforeseen' proteins that are created during the mixing of the genes of different plants and bacteria's have been proven to be allergenic and toxic to animals and humans and pass this damaging genetic material to the bacteria in your gut which alters them in a negative way.

This coupled with the herbicide 'Glyphosate' that is sprayed on them damages and alters the gut biome further.

It is important to know that in the US, literally all processed foods contain GMO crops.

Dairy – We are seeing across the world more and more people becoming 'lactose intolerant' which means their gut is not handling dairy very well. With the consumption of dairy, we are seeing the increase of bad bacteria in the gut that leads to inflammation and damage.

This coupled with the fact that dairy is very mucus forming and as such lines the tract and can make it

128

harder for nutrients to be absorbed all makes a difference in how our gut functions.

Again, it is important to further point out that most people who consume dairy today are not consuming organic and raw dairy, but instead are consuming the mass produced cheap dairy. These animals are fed on GMO feed and so the milk that is consumed from them will indeed contain these GMO allergenic proteins which, as we have mentioned, damage the gut and alter the gut biome.

Cheap meats – This comes down to the same point as mentioned above. Animals used in factory farming, which is the majority of meat on the market for sale, in restaurants, fast foods chains, processed foods etc are fed with GMO feed that stays in the animals meat until it is consumed by a person. This is true for a wide range of countries including across the EU too.

Gluten – As we are seeing more and more, people are becoming intolerant to gluten which is found in wheat, barley, rye and spelt. This is because the gluten molecule is very hard to digest and has been found to cause damage to the lining of the gut that can lead to damaged villi (the hair like protrusions in the gut that absorb nutrients into the body) and a 'leaky gut' which can lead to autoimmune diseases, allergies and neurological disorders. This is also what 'Celiacs Disease' is.

Sugar - Sugar feeds the bad bacteria in the gut and can contribute to overgrowth of 'Candida' which too can damage the gut and cause it to become permeable. For this reason, sugar should be reduced if not eliminated from the diet altogether (some fruits will still be ok as these come with a range of nutrients, antioxidants and fibre that is good for the body). This will include foods that turn to sugar too like wheat and anything made with wheat (which falls under the gluten label), white rice, white potatoes and other such starchy foods.

Toxic Chemical Exposure – Toxic chemicals, especially 'neurotoxins' are very damaging to the nervous system and can alter the way in which the neurones communicate with each other. (We will get into the specific ones and where they can be found in the solutions section).

Medications are also something to be considered, especially antibiotics.

Antibiotics actually alter the functioning of the gut biome too by destroying bacteria. Not only that, but the antibiotics can actually make the bad bacteria in the gut stronger and can make them resistant to these medications, which will make situations in the gut even worse in the long run.

Other medications such as antacids and anti-inflammatories will also cause more harm than good as antacids will stop the sufficient production of stomach acid and as such will reduce its ability of breaking everything down properly which increases the chances of harmful bacteria and undigested proteins getting through into the blood stream, such as leaky gut, and anti-inflammatories will artificially reduce inflammation, which is incidentally the immune response to damage in the body, and so will allow the 'attack' that the immune system was reacting to in the gut to continue.

Next, Glutathione

Glutathione, which we have mentioned a few times through out this book, is the body's most powerful antioxidant and the production of this enzyme is actually impaired in those with autism. As it is the body's most powerful antioxidant, when it is impaired in this way, heavy metals, free radicals and other environmental toxins can build up in the system and contribute to its hastened malfunctioning and deterioration.

Finally, vaccines can indeed be a cause of Autism.

As you would have read in the 'Whistle blowers' part of the 'Understanding The Epidemic' section, when these aborted fetal cells are used in vaccine production, they have the ability to cause negative reactions in the body and thus neurological difficulties such as Autism and autoimmune responses can indeed develop from their exposure.

If you have not read that section yet, please be sure to, especially the testimony from 'Dr. Deisher' who has spent many years working with fetal cells and has lots of experience in the matter.

You may have heard that there is a genetic component to Autism, and that is true. This is because the parents can already have these factors mentioned above happening within their system to some degree and as such pass these on to the unborn baby which you can see develop in their young age whilst their immune system, body and organs are still trying to develop.

So as you can see the causes to Autism all come about when unnatural alterations happen in the system. As we all know, the internal environment of the body is paramount to good health.

Symptoms

There can be a wide range of symptoms for autism and people on the autism spectrum. These can include some core symptoms such as problems with eye to eye contact, unresponsive facial expressions, withdrawn from interacting with other people, can have lack of empathy, difficulty with understanding, speech and learning.

Solutions

The solution to Autism comprises of healing the gut, ensuring there is good nutrition to the brain, removing already accumulated toxins and allergens and ensuring no more enter the system, utilizing plenty of antioxidants and stimulating the release of the neurotransmitter oxytocin.

Healing the gut

First and foremost, we must ensure to restore the balance of good to bad bacteria, reduce any inflammation that may be present and heal any permeability that may be allowing undigested proteins into the blood.

As we have listed this in great detail under the 'Leaky Gut' section of this book, please be sure to have a look at that to begin working to heal the gut.

By healing the gut properly, neurotransmitters such as Serotonin and others can then start to do their job again sufficiently.

Nutrition to the brain
Next, or simultaneously, we want to ensure we are healing and giving the correct nutrition to the brain as during the process of the gut becoming damaged, the brain will be too.

This is also the reason for brain fog when the gut is inflamed because there is inflammation present in the brain too.

If you are sure to include the foods we mention in the 'Body Essentials' part of this book under 'Foods containing the amino acids, fats, carbohydrates, minerals and vitamins the body needs', these will give the brain all it needs to function fully and at its optimum level. This list also contains a range of antioxidants, toxin detoxifiers and the essential raw materials the body needs to be at its best.

Removing toxins and allergens from the system
Again, simultaneously, we want to ensure we are clearing out already accumulated toxins and known allergens that will slow our progress in moving forward.

As we mentioned in the causes section, this will be things such as GMO foods (and cheap meats), dairy products, foods containing gluten and medications such as antibiotics and others that will add further complications to the gut biome. We also want to ensure we reduce our exposure to toxic substances such as processed foods, junk foods, fried foods, fizzy drinks, drinks containing artificial colours and sweeteners, foods and drinks containing preservatives, further vaccinations, unfiltered water and other such things that are not conducive to a healthy and strong functioning nervous and immune system and body as a whole.

Instead what we want to replace these substances with are nutrient rich, natural and whole foods such as an abundance of fresh and organic vegetables (especially dark leafy greens), fresh and organic fruit (both vegetables and fruits contain a wide range of vitamins and minerals that are essential for nervous and immune system health and functioning), sufficient amounts of clean protein as the amino acids present are very important (clean protein meaning not from the sources mentioned above of processed and junk foods etc) and sufficient amounts of saturated fats like coconut oil and omega 3 fatty acids (for healthy cell membrane building).

Increasing intake of antioxidants
Whilst the foods mentioned in the 'Foods containing the amino acids, fats, carbohydrates, minerals and vitamins the body needs' contain a wide range of antioxidants, there are some in specific you may want to increase. These are things such as:

Whole foods containing vitamin c, vitamin e, selenium (acts as a precursor to glutathione), glutathione supplementation, whole foods containing resveratrol such as red grapes and raw cocoa, curcumin found in turmeric root, blueberries and other berries, nuts, dark leafy greens like kale and other greens and green tea.

All of these will offset the oxidative stress and free radical damage that can happen across the nervous system and to other cells all over the body too.

Finally, a few last things to consider would be:

- Moving away from the factors we discussed in the 'so, what causes it?' section
- Increase levels of vitamin d in the system, if supplementing it may be best to use vitamin d3
- Ensure to get a good amount of all the essential amino acids (protein) as these are definitely needed for assisting the body in recovering

You can use these suggestions as a starting point and I hope this will spur you on to look deeper into the things we mentioned here to help in working with autism.

Bad Breath

What is it?
While not a disease in and of itself, persistent bad breath can be a sign of something else happening in the body.

Kind of self-explanatory, but bad breath refers to continuous and persistent foul smelling breath. In severe cases this can be referred to as 'Halitosis'.

So, what causes it?
There could be a range of causes for bad breath, such as:

- Bad or insufficient digestion (such as from poor stomach acid causing acid reflux)
- Excessive bacterial growth in the mouth
- Poor oral hygiene
- 'Candida' overgrowth in the GI tract and mouth (which is a fungal overgrowth)
- Gum disease
- Unclean tongue - which actually relates to toxin accumulation or other issues with internal organs depending on the state of the tongue and which part of the tongue is affected - this is something that is very well known in 'Traditional Chinese Medicine' and the Indian practice of 'Ayurveda'
- Dry mouth - which can be from lack of sufficient fluid intake or can indicate a problem with the kidneys but also can be from a range of medications if the person is taking any, infections, excessive alcohol intake and

smoking.

So there really are a wide range of causes for having bad breath.

Symptoms
The symptom of bad breath is well... bad smelling breath.

Solutions
As there are so many potential causes for bad breath, we have areas of this book that can help you address the potential different causes of it.

If the bad breath comes from an issue of poor digestion which can be characterised by lots of burping, acid reflux and bloating, it would be advisable to view our 'Acid Reflux' page to see how to rectify that problem.

If it is down to a fungal overgrowth problem, which can be characterised by increasing fungal infections of the skin and nails, lots of white 'fur' on the tongue, bad sugar cravings and thrush see our 'Candida' page to see how to rectify that problem and also be sure to read our 'Gum Disease' page to see how to rectify that condition and keep the teeth and gums healthy.

Before checking out those pages to help with bad breath, there are some general things you can try such as:

- Using a tongue scraper and cleaning the tongue when you brush your teeth to clean off the bacterial growth (but remember the tongue is a mirror of the internal organs in the body and so should be looked at in a deeper way)

- Drink plenty of fresh and filtered water and eat foods that hydrate the body and avoid foods and drinks that dehydrate the body and suck nutrients out of the system (processed foods, junk foods, fatty foods, fried foods, chemically filled foods, caffeine, alcohol, fizzy drinks and such)

- Cut down on eating foods high in sugar and foods high in carbohydrates as these will actually fuel the bacterial and/or fungal growth in the GI tract

It will be very beneficial to eat foods such as celery, watermelon, cucumber and iceberg lettuce and other fresh, organic and raw fruits and vegetables to keep the body hydrated and topped up on the essential minerals and vitamins that help to fight off bad bacteria and infections. It is advisable to have more vegetables than fruit in this case though due to the sugars in the fruit.

Be sure to check out those pages we mentioned above and put these into a workable strategy and you will notice a marked difference in bad breath.

Bronchitis

What is it?
Bronchitis is a condition in which the lining of the bronchial tubes become infected and inflamed which causes the person affected to have excessive mucus in the tubes.

This condition along with 'Emphysema' and 'Asthma' contribute to the condition known as 'COPD - Chronic Obstructive Pulmonary Disorder' which generally just refers to a range of conditions that block airflow and make it difficult for the person affected to breathe.

So, what causes it?
Well this condition comes down to the bronchial tubes of the lungs being damaged and so when we think of this condition we must look at things such as mould exposure, smoking, continuous exposure to fumes and air pollution, second hand smoke exposure, history of lung infections, harmful chemicals and toxins in the system, and (as with many breathing conditions) damage to the nervous system especially around C1, C2 and C3. C standing for 'Cervical' which is the top portion of the spine.

This area of the nervous system controls the diaphragm and so controls the breathing too.

Symptoms
Symptoms can include chesty, deep cough that persists, lots of mucus and phlegm creation, pain or tenderness in the chest while coughing, shortness of

breath, wheezing and feeling tired. Some people can also get a fever when they have this condition, but not all.

Solutions

The solutions are based around utilising foods that strengthen and cleanse mucus out of the lungs and methods to strengthen the nervous and immune system.

So the suggestions here would be to:

- Drink lots of fresh and filtered water

- Consume lots of fresh and organic orange and yellow fruit and veg (as these contain beta-carotene which is great for lung health when eaten from natural sources, not supplemental beta-carotene).

> Foods high in beta-carotene are things such as carrots, melons, mangos, apricots, squash, peppers and sweet potatoes but also leafy greens like spinach, kale and greens.

Other methods are going to include deep breathing to get the most amount of oxygen into the system as possible. Deep breathing also helps to stimulate the lymphatic system to help remove waste from cells and tissues.

Doing deep breathing over a steaming bowl of water with a few drops of tea tree oil in is going to be a great way to really clear the lungs of mucus, remove any bacterial build up and help increase oxygen intake.

We also want to boost the immune system through things such as regular exercise (not doing more than you can manage, but just enough to keep the body moving and stop blood flow from stagnating), proper nutrition and eliminating toxins out of the system.

With regards to toxins, stressors and irritants to the immune system we would recommend you read our 'Holistic Immune System Building' section where we have detailed are range of ways in which to deal with these and strengthen this system.

Instead of us trying to include all of the things that need to be considered with regards to having a healthy and strong nervous system, we have put all of the detail into the 'Holistic Nervous System Building' section of this book so please be sure to have a read of that too.

I will, however, mention here that we want to avoid neurotoxins.

Some of the most harmful neurotoxins to be aware of are things like:

- Fluoride (which is found in many toothpastes, mouthwashes and water supplies)
- Pesticides, Herbicides and Fungicides (sprayed on literally all food crops)
- MSG (Monosodium Glutamate - found in a wide range of foods - as a note, anything that says 'Flavouring' but is not defined as exactly what that is, could very much be MSG)

- Aspartame and Sucralose (which are artificial sweeteners found in many foods and drinks - read ALL of your food labels - especially those things that say 'diet' and 'sugar free')
- Aluminium (a heavy metal found in vaccines, drinking water and medications)
- Mercury (a heavy metal which can be found in water, fish products, vaccines and tooth fillings)

As well as addressing the nervous system and the immune system, here are some additional factors to bear in mind and implement:

Posture: It is important to have good posture as when we are misaligned in the way we sit, walk and stand, the nerves are also misaligned and stressed and so do not function to their fullest capacity. Try to keep the neck, spine and head aligned as much as you can.

Mucus Forming Foods: Eliminate mucus forming foods such as dairy, fatty, inorganic meats and other acidic food (another reason why we recommend fresh, organic and preferably raw fruits and vegetables, especially dark leafy greens in abundance), avoid soy and cut down on grains like white rice and especially those containing gluten like wheat, barley and rye.

Mucus Clearing: Mucus clearing and anti-inflammatory foods and substances are going include pumpkin seeds, ginger, onions, garlic, honey, pineapple and grapefruit. Foods high in omega-3 fatty acids (such as krill oil, algae oils, ground chia and flax seeds and seaweed such as kelp) and Vitamins A, C, D and E + Selenium will be of great use. Also ensure to include lots of dark leafy greens and fresh and filtered water. Juicing and blending is a great way to get the greens into your system.

Remember to have the foods organic and as fresh and as raw as possible for the greatest effects.

Please be sure to read our 'Holistic Nervous System Building' and 'Holistic Immune System Building' sections of this book too.

Cardiovascular Disease

What is it?
Cardiovascular disease can include a wide range of ailments that essentially restrict, obstruct or alter the functioning of the heart, arteries and vessels that take blood around the body.

Problems can be with the heart muscle itself such as rhythm problems and problems with the values, problems with the arteries, problems with blood vessels and other related issues.

So, what causes it?
So, now we have established exactly what it is, we can address the causes much better.

When we look at the arteries of the body, we can see that if there are any problems here then the heart and circulation is going to be affected. Vitamin C deficiency can actually cause cracks in the artery walls, so this is something that can be a cause.

Another problem is calcification of the artery walls (atherosclerosis) which can be caused by damage of the interior walls of the arteries and plaque build-up.

Factors such as smoking, high levels of LDL cholesterol in the blood (which, incidentally, is trying to help heal the body), high blood pressure (which deteriorates the inside lining, amongst over things) and high blood sugar will affect the arteries and heart.

One of the leading causes of death in the western

world is heart disease. So we must consider the food that we are consuming as a cause of this.

The west has very high levels of fat, sugar and salt in the diet, high amounts of chemicals in the foods and drinks and lots of processed and junk foods.

All of these affect the cardiovascular system in a negative way and can lead to heart disease.

Other factors that can lead to cardiovascular disease are:

- A lack of exercise which causes blood and fluids to stagnate which forces the heart to work harder

- Unhealthy lungs and poor oxygen intake which increases carbon dioxide levels as thus increases the blood pressure

- Being overweight which puts pressure on the heart and causes plaques to build up in the arteries

- Long use of medications as it can deplete the body of its natural enzymes, water and oxygen which will again make the heart have to work harder and increase the blood pressure amongst other things

- The body being in a continuously stressed state as this raises the blood pressure, blood sugar, cholesterol levels and releases stress hormones such as cortisol which if sustained at high levels for long periods of time can be damaging to the cardiovascular system.

This will then reduce the level of repair that happens in the body and the amount of oxygen circulated.

- High intake of sugar as this can damage the artery walls. This will then call more LDL cholesterol into the blood which can lead to plaque build-up and then hardening of the arteries (Atherosclerosis)

Medications such as blood pressure lowering medications can actually be dangerous for the cardiovascular system as they artificially lower the blood pressure which the body has raised in order to get blood to where it is needed. Prolonged use of these can cause more damage.

It is better to address the core problem of what is causing the rise in blood pressure. Of course, I do not recommend just coming off of medications without working with a healthcare professional. These types of medications are actually very important if your life is at risk without them, so never, ever just stop taking any medications 'cold turkey'.

Symptoms
Symptoms can include chest pain, shortness of breath, numbness or coldness in arms and legs, aches and pains in the body, arrhythmia (irregular heart beat), dizziness, lightheaded and possible fainting.

Solutions

We have to remember the body does what it does to adapt to the environment which we have created within it. For this reason we should be aware of this and act accordingly, not just act to suppress or address the symptoms, but try to understand what is happening in the body that has caused these symptoms.

With that in mind, here are a few things that would be advisable to do to reduce the continued impact of those factors which have caused the range of problems that is cardiovascular disease.

It would be advisable to implement things such as:

- Reducing intake of sugar, especially refined and added sugars

- Reducing intake of trans-fats and hydrogenated oils found in junk and processed foods

- Reducing mucus causing foods such as dairy and fatty meats

- Help reduce high blood pressure by eating lots of fresh, organic and raw fruit and vegetables (especially dark leafy greens). This will also help to start breaking down any plaque build ups in the arteries too

- Have a good intake of daily Vitamin C which will help to boost the immune system and repair the lining of the arteries

- Ensuring not to add more chemicals into the system through things like smoking and drinking alcohol

- Reduce fatty meats such as red meat and animal proteins (but make no mistake, you still need to get the sufficient amount of amino acids into your system to stay healthy, just cutting out protein from animals and not replacing it with the amino acids found in plants will not suffice). This is recommended because these can turn acidic in the system after being consumed

- Keep the body moving, even if it is light exercise such as walking which will help to keep the lymphatic system working and the blood flowing sufficiently

- Practice deep, abdominal breathing to ensure a sufficient amount of oxygen gets into the system

- Ensure to not consume GMO foods

Remember our 'Body Essentials' section of the book? Put the foods mentioned here into your plans to ensure the body gets all that it needs.

If you have not read it yet, I would recommend you do so. Essentially, it details that the best combination of foods for you to consume are organic, fresh and predominantly raw and fall into the categories of fruits, vegetables, seeds, nuts and good fats.

Putting all of these points into practice in daily life will indeed improve the condition of cardiovascular disease.

Cancer

What is it?
Putting it into simple terms, cancer is the condition whereby cells become abnormal and start to multiply uncontrollably. This generally happens because the cells have been damaged or altered in some way.

The cells lose their ability of 'apoptosis' also known as 'programmed cell death' which is the ability of damaged cells or cells that have been changed to self-destruct as to not cause problems to surrounding cells and tissues. When this apoptosis does not happen, the proliferation of the damaged cell begins. As this builds up, they form tumours. These cells can then move to other parts of the body and stop in new places. When they do this, a process called 'angiogenesis' then occurs.

Angiogenesis is essentially when the faulty cells send out chemical signals that tell nearby cells to do the same and grow new blood vessels that can feed the faulty cells and thus proliferate the tumour. Some cancerous cells can also produce their own growth hormone and proliferate that way.

So, what causes it?
Well we have established that cancer is abnormal or damaged cells that start to proliferate. So, what can cause cells to become damaged in the first place? Let's start there.

Harmful Chemicals

So, first and foremost, harmful chemicals and toxins must be explored. Before we get into those chemicals, let just talk about why these may cause cancerous cell growth.

It is known that harmful and synthetic chemicals interfere with the cells ability to communicate efficiently with each other.

These synthetic chemicals can displace other bio-chemicals and enzymes that the body needs to function properly (as an example, the synthetic chemical fluoride in the body will displace iodine, which is a very important substance for the thyroid and metabolism of bodily processes).

Synthetic chemicals can also cause the body to be leached of vitamins and minerals. This happens because with the introduction of synthetic chemicals comes lots of free radicals. These then have to be eliminated by using the body's natural antioxidants. This means that the vitamins and minerals in the body get used up at a much faster rate which will deplete the body of what it needs to stay healthy and disease free.

We must understand that cells use the raw materials we give them to create new cells.

If the body is full of chemicals and depleted of the vitamins and minerals it needs to create healthy new cells, then the body will use what it has available to build the new cells. It is then obvious to see why abnormal cells can be created in this environment and why, with an abundance of chemicals in the system, cells can become damaged easily.

Within this class of harmful synthetic chemicals are also 'Neurotoxins'. These are toxic chemicals that affect the cells of the nervous system by disrupting the communication and processing of the cells and can even cause death of the neurones.

When the electrical communication of the body starts to break down, so does everything else.

Some of the most harmful neurotoxins to avoid are:

- Fluoride (which is found in many toothpastes, mouthwashes and water supplies)
- Pesticides (sprayed on literally all crops)
- Herbicides and Fungicides (also sprayed on most crops)
- MSG (Monosodium Glutamate - found in a wide range of foods - as a note, anything that says 'Flavouring' but is not defined as exactly what it is could very much be MSG)
- Aspartame and Sucralose (which are artificial sweeteners found in many foods and drinks - read ALL of your food labels - especially those things that say 'diet' and 'sugar free')
- Aluminium (found in vaccines, drinking water and medications)
- Mercury (which can be found in water, fish products, vaccines and tooth fillings)

These are all very important, so the way we have listed these are not in order of importance.

Radiation
The next thing that can alter the healthy growth of

cells is harmful radiation which can also create an internal environment that is conducive for cancerous cells to grow and proliferate. This can come from excessive UV rays, medical procedures such as CT Scans, X-Rays and MRIs (which is why these things have a limit of the number that can be had in one year), continuous aeroplane flights (but you would have to be literally flying all the time).

These radiation sources alone do not cause much harm, but with repeated and frequent exposure they could possibly contribute to the damage of cells so it is something that should still be considered.

Harmful chemicals, neurotoxins and radiation can all contribute to genetic changes too which can cause cancer to come about.

Congestions
Next up we have congestions in the body in the form of excessive fat, clogged arteries and veins and traumas to the body which can cause cells to become stagnant, which stops oxygen and nutrients getting to the area and when this happens the potential for cells to become damaged increases. This then increases the ability for cancerous cells to form and grow.

Acidic Blood pH
An acidic body is definitely a cause for concern in cancer development.

The body is naturally at a slightly alkaline state (7.4pH) when healthy. If the body drops below this (becomes more acidic) then oxygen levels fall, mineral and vitamin assimilation is not as efficient and cancer has the perfect opportunity to develop in this environment.

We will detail how diet can affect your blood pH in the solutions section.

Genetically Modified Organism's (GMOs)
GMO foods are crops that have been genetically altered in a lab. Generally, the seeds have been altered to express desirable traits and this is done by taking the DNA from one plant, bacteria or something similar and mixing that with the DNA of another plant.

For example, plants that have been genetically altered to produce their own pesticides from within so that any bug that tries to eat or that touches the plant will receive a dose of harmful chemical that is designed to rupture its stomach and kill it.

The altering of the food chain in this way is actually untested over long periods for human consumption. Never the less, it continues to be added to our foods that most people consume.

As you would have seen in our 'Understanding the Epidemic' section of this book, the correlation between the increases of GMO foods in our food chain and cancer and other disease rates have been increasing together.

Now of course correlation does not always equal causation, but knowing that these foods were untested for safe human consumption before they were put out into the market, and knowing that the animal models that have been subjected to the GMO foods and the powerful pesticides and herbicides that go with these have seen significant negative results when tested for longer than 3 months, is it worth the risk?

As an additional point, some of these plants have been modified to be able to still grow whilst being subjected to very strong pesticide and herbicide chemicals such as Glyphosate (known as 'Round-Up'). This kills literally all other weeds, bugs and other living organisms around the plant.

So not only are we consuming altered foods that seem to have a negative effect on the human organism, but we are also subjected to even stronger, more harmful and more toxic pest and herbicidess that are sprayed on these plants. Residues then stay on the plants and enter into our bodies when we consume these.

GMO foods are predominantly found in processed and junk foods, although they are banned in the EU to be used directly in products, there is no such ban in the US.

Russia has now ban all GMO food crops and anyone caught growing them is automatically fined for it. China have also started rejecting large amounts of GMO exports from the US of these crops.

Important note about GM foods: While there may be bans on GMO foods used in direct products in Europe, these GMO crops are allowed to be used as animal feed which then come to make up the animal and then of course people eat them. This means that people who do not think they are exposed to GMO foods directly are indeed consuming GMO foods through eating meat and consuming dairy that is not grass fed and raised organically.

This is a very important point that should be considered. This is always the reason why you should never consume cheap, factory farmed meats. Only organic, grass fed, lean meats and organic and raw dairy.

Finally, sugar
Sugar and foods that turn to sugar will feed cancer and in high amounts, mixed with an acidic diet, will drastically increase the chances of developing cancer. It is literally that simple. Sugar feeds cancer development and deteriorates the body.

Symptoms
Possible symptoms can include problems with going to the toilet, finding lumps around the body, lumps increasing in size/tenderness/pain, unexplained weight loss, changes in skin, fever and fatigue, unusual bleeding and continuous hoarse cough.

Solutions
First and foremost, we must give the body the raw materials it needs to build healthy new cells and we must focus on fortifying the immune system which has the ability to destroy cancerous cells itself.

These raw materials for building cells can be obtained

from the diet and to see how we can fortify and rebuild the immune system, please visit our 'Holistic Immune System Building' section of this book where we have gone into detail about this.

The body needs healthy 'good' fats which make up the outer lining of the cells and helps with the incoming and outgoing messages of the cell.

These fats are contained in things such as olives, avocados, coconut oil, oily fish and fish oils, algae oils, seaweed, ground chia and flax seeds, hemp seeds, sunflower seeds and other seeds, pecans, walnuts, almonds and other nuts.

Saturated fats are important for the healthy functioning of the cells and more than enough can be obtained from coconut oil which is predominantly saturated fat. The bonus of using coconut oil over other sources is that it also comes with a wide range of healing and rejuvenating properties.

Next, the body uses amino acids to build new cells. How do we get amino acids? The proteins we consume get broken down by the stomach acid into the individual amino acids. They then pass through the intestines where they are absorbed and used by the body.

To ensure we are getting the amino acids we need, we must ensure that the stomach acid and GI tract are healthy so that we are breaking down and absorbing them. To do this we need to ensure we are not deficient in Vitamin b1, zinc, iodine and salt and that the blood is not in too much of an acidic state in order to have sufficient stomach acid to break down the food (more on this in the 'Acid Reflux' section) and secondly we need to ensure the GI Tract is not inflamed and it is strong so that the nutrients can be absorbed (more on this in the 'Leaky Gut' section).

Healthy sources of protein can be found in nuts, seeds, beans and grains (brown rice and quinoa).

Other types of foods that should be consumed are fresh, organic and predominantly raw dark leafy greens such as kale, collard, turnip, mustard and burdock greens, swiss chard and spinach. If you put these into juices and blends it makes it much easier for the body to digest and assimilate the nutrients from them.

Also a range of fresh, organic and raw fruits and vegetables should be the predominant diet to be consumed to help balance the body and get as much nutrients and enzymes in as possible (more vegetables than fruits as cancer thrives on sugar, although there are some low sugar fruits such as lemons and limes).

We also want to cleanse excessive mucus out of the body. Excessive mucus can cause stagnation in the system and when this happens bacteria has a chance to grow and thrive, which will put even more tax on the immune system in having to deal with these issues and in these areas cancerous cells can also accumulate and proliferate.

So, we can eliminate excessive mucus by, first and foremost, cutting out mucus forming foods such as diary, fatty meats, yeast, sugar (and anything that turns to sugar such as wheat, white rice, white potatoes and other starchy foods) and anything else that is acidic.

To help dissolve the already accumulated mucus in the system it is advisable to consume things such as cayenne pepper (which actually can help combat the cancer too in some cases), garlic and onions, foods high in iodine, pumpkin seeds, pineapple (not in high amounts due to its sugar content), ginger and, again, lots of fresh and organic fruit and vegetables (especially dark leafy greens).

Staying with the idea of cleansing, we also want to eliminate toxins and chemicals that we consume in the foods and drinks we have, products that we use (for body and home) and the ones that have already accumulated in the body to ensure no obstructions are reducing the body's natural ability to function at its fullest capacity.

You also want to drink lots of fresh and filtered water and ensure to do as much exercise as you can as even light exercise, such as walking, is very good for stimulating the lymphatic system and ensuring oxygen continues to circulate properly.

Specific things with regards to cancer that should be considered to take are:

Curcumin. This is the active ingredient in turmeric root which has been shown to be able to kill cancer cells and stop more from growing and spreading.

A real super spice that has anti-inflammatory, anti-bacterial and rejuvenating effects too.

Hemp Oil. Hemp oil or cannabis oil has had thousands of testimonials from people who were suffering from cancer reporting that they eradicated the disease by taking cannabis oil.

Studies have found that cancerous cells in culture have reacted very well to cannabis oil by killing the cancerous cells by triggering 'apoptosis' (or programmed cell death), preventing blood vessels from fuelling tumours, stopping cells from dividing and stopping the spreading of the cancerous cells.

It should be noted that these results are from using THC and CBD from the oil and that these were studies done in culture, which means on cells outside of the body.

Resveratrol. Resveratrol is an antioxidant and powerful compound found in red grapes (the skins), raw cocoa, peanuts and some berries. It is also found in large amounts in red wine, but you do not want to put alcohol in your system when you have cancer at all.

Resveratrol has been shown to be able to get into the heart of the cell and help with repairs and protect from cancerous developments.

While being able to help with the management of cancer it has also been shown to be very good at offsetting some of the nasty side effects of pharmaceutical drugs used in the treatment of cancer as well.

Mind set. Your mind set and mental structure is very

important and contributes significantly to your health and wellbeing. We could do an entire book on this subject itself, but it is enough to say that being in a stressful state from negative thinking, anger, worry, anxiety, stress and other negative emotional states will cause chemical reactions to happen in your body that can actually make the body toxic, run down and suppress the immune system and so it will have a reduced ability to protect you from disease and infections.

This will then contribute to cell damage and problems in the system.

In a case such as cancer where we need the immune system to be functioning at its very best to help us eradicate the problem, a negative mind set is actually going to work against us and make it much harder for the body to heal.

Try your very best to de-stress yourself through things such as meditation, yoga, light exercise, listening to relaxing music, getting out in nature and other such things.

Blood pH. How does your diet change your blood pH?

First and foremost, the stomach must be at a certain pH to digest food. Depending on the food that goes into the stomach, this will determine the reaction that must take place.

In order to lower the stomachs pH to the level where food can be digested, when food enters the stomach, hydrochloric acid is secreted to lower that pH. As this happens, the same amount of sodium bicarbonate is secreted into the blood which helps to keep the body slightly alkaline.

When we eat acidic foods, the amount of hydrochloric acid needed to be secreted to get the pH low enough to break up the food is not that much meaning that not much sodium bicarbonate will be secreted into the blood either. If a diet is continued in this way, then the body will struggle to keep the blood pH in the slightly alkaline state of 7.4pH.

On the other hand, if we eat alkaline foods such as most fruits and lots of vegetables the body has to secrete lots of hydrochloric acid in order to get the pH low enough to break down the food. This means that lots of sodium bicarbonate will also be secreted into the blood and this will make it a lot easier for the body to maintain its slightly alkaline state.

For this reason, and a host of other reasons, eating alkaline foods such as a range of fruits and vegetables is very good for the body and blood in its attempt to stay strong, vibrant and healthy. Remember though, also have lots more vegetables than fruits because of the sugar in fruits. In moderate amounts this is ok, but we do not want to have too much sugar entering the system at this time.

Go through this section a few times and read over all of the things we have mentioned here. Those who are suffering with cancer, implementing these things will definitely help you in dealing with the condition and for those worried about cancer, these points mentioned are powerful preventative measures that you can take to stay clear of the disease.

Candida

What is it?

Candida is a fungal yeast that is naturally present in the body. When we talk about Candida, we are generally referring to the overgrowth of this yeast that grows in the intestinal tract. If it continues to grow uninterrupted, problems such as nutritional deficiencies, allergies, fatigue and range of other issues that stem from poor gut health can happen due to the fungal overgrowth covering and damaging the intestinal tract which stops the sufficient absorption of nutrients into the system.

So, what causes it?

The cause of candida overgrowth is things like having lots of sugar in the diet as it grows on sugar. Having too much sugar in the diet also lowers the immune system and so gives the yeast more time to grow uninterrupted.

Most medications can also cause problems as they are toxic, especially antibiotics, which damage the good bacteria in the gut which help to keep the candida in check.

So anything else that damages good bacteria and promotes bad bacterial growth will also allow candida to grow. This can be from processed and junk foods, un-organic and non grass fed meats and dairy, alcohol, stress and an acidic diet too.

Symptoms

Some of the symptoms can include fatigue, weight gain, gas, joint pain, bad breath, bloating and white 'fur' on the tongue.

Solutions

Definitely avoid sugar causing foods. This would be foods with added sugar and foods that turn to sugar such as white potatoes, white rice, wheat and other starchy foods.

Avoid things that can destroy and alter the good bacteria in the gut. Acidic foods such as fizzy drinks, processed foods, junk foods, dairy (mucus forming), caffeine, fatty, cheap meats (which contain GMOs), alcohol, gluten, stressful situations and other such things will cause damage to the intestines. Medications can also do this, so it is best to avoid medications where possible, especially antibiotics.

The other thing that can damage the gut is chemicals and neurotoxins in the, again, processed and junks foods, unfiltered water and household cleaning and hygiene products we use.

Beneficial things would be to eat lots of fresh, organic and raw vegetables, especially dark leafy greens and reduce fruit intake too as these contain sugar also. Once the candida is in check you can return to eating fresh fruit. You can juice and blend the vegetables to make it easier for the body to assimilate the nutrients from it also.

Do what you can to keep the body out of a stressed state. This includes chemical, emotional and physical stresses.

This is because when the body is in a stressed state, stress hormones are elevated and this elevates the blood pressure, elevates the blood sugar, suppresses the immune system and keeps the body in the sympathetic nervous system state, known as the 'fight or flight' response.

In order to heal and get blood flow and energy back to the gut, we need to get the body into the parasympathetic nervous system state, known as the 'rest and digest' state, and we do this by ensuring we keep chemical, emotional and physical stressors to a minimum.

In order to repopulate the good bacteria in the gut it may also be a good idea to take and consume probiotics. This can be in supplemental form or from sources such as fermented vegetables like sauerkraut.

Celiac Disease

What is it?

Celiac disease in simple terms is a reaction to gluten in which the gluten molecule causes inflammation and the destruction of the tiny hair like 'villi' which are located on the inside lining of the intestines. These villi are responsible for absorbing the nutrients from your food that are broken down in the stomach and pass through into the intestines.

When this problem occurs, getting nutrients into the system then becomes an issue and can present a range of additional complications such as nutritional deficiencies amongst other things. This can then lead to something called 'Leaky Gut' and we have put that in its own section in this book.

Essentially though this means that the permeability of the lining of the gut becomes compromised from things such as the inflammation and breaking down of villi. Undigested proteins can then slip through the gaps and enter straight into the blood stream which the body sees as foreign and mounts an attack against it.

In the 'Leaky Gut' section of this book you will see how this can lead to autoimmune diseases as well, which celiac disease is classed as.

So, what causes it?

A gluten intolerance causes this condition in which the gut reacts to its presence. That is the cause of celiac disease. Gluten is found in wheat, barley, rye, spelt and foods made with/containing any amount of these. Another factor which increases the chances of developing celiac disease can be due to genetics.

Symptoms
Symptoms can include problems with digestion such as bloating, pain and excessive gas, diarrhoea, weight loss, rashes, joint pain, cramps and a wide range of other issues due to malnutrition as the villi become damaged and stop absorbing the nutrients.

Solutions
First and foremost, it is important to cut gluten out from the diet completely and that includes all foods that are made with anything containing gluten which is wheat, barley, rye and spelt. This will stop the reaction from happening which will stop further inflammation and destruction of the villi.

This will then give you a chance to try and heal the gut that has been damaged. As this falls directly under the 'Leaky Gut' process, please see the 'Leaky Gut' section of this book to see how to heal this condition.

In most cases, as long as the damage is not too extensive, the inflammation will subside and the villi will actually grow back and health can return to normal.

Crohn's Disease

What is it?

Crohn's disease is a chronic condition whereby the intestines become inflamed and it is considered an 'auto-immune' disease which essentially means that the body is attacking itself. In this case it is attacking the intestines and that can be anywhere from the mouth to the end of the colon. It can then cause ulcers, erosion of the intestine walls, scaring in the intestines which will also stop it from working properly and can narrow the intestines which can cause food to get caught there leading to pain and cramping.

So, what causes it?

As this relates to the intestines, we have to consider the elements that can damage this area. We must also remember that 80% of the immune system is located in our gut.

If there happens to be an over powering of bad bacteria over our good bacteria in the gut, viruses, parasites or infections present in other areas of the body, this can reduce the effectiveness of our immune system in keeping the body healthy and as such damage can accumulate which can lead to inflammation.

As we will learn in the 'Leaky Gut' section of this book, damage in the gut can lead to autoimmune diseases and other allergic reactions.

These factors, bad bacteria build up, viruses, parasites and infections, can come about through not giving the body the right nutrients it needs to stay healthy and eating the wrong foods which will increase the amount of bad bacteria in the gut.

This damage and inflammation to the gut can also be caused by chemical accumulations in the form of medications, especially things like antibiotics, anti-inflammatories and also antacids. Antibiotics can break down and kill the good bacteria of the gut which helps to keep it healthy. Anti-inflammatories can artificially reduce the inflammation of the gut, which is actually the body attempting to heal itself, which will then allow the original problem to persist and not address the cause.

Finally, antacids will cause the stomach acid to be diluted, which will cause the food coming into the system to not be digested properly and any harmful bacteria's to not be disposed of fully in the stomach acid.

Symptoms

Depending on the area affected, different symptoms can be presented. For example 'Crohn's Colitis' is inflammation of just the colon, 'Crohn's Enteritis' is inflammation in the small intestines and 'Crohn's Ileitis' is inflammation of the bottom half of the small intestines just before it joins up with the colon (large intestine). Symptoms then can vary between fever, weight loss, nausea, vomiting, fatigue, growth issues, rectal bleeding and psychological problems too.

Solutions

Firstly, while it may reduce your symptoms in the initial period of time, it is best to try and avoid pharmaceutical drugs that just cover up or suppress the symptoms as these can cause more problems in the long run and will contribute to gut damage.

It is important to have good hydration of fresh and filtered water (not distilled water, as distilled water actually sucks the nutrients out of your system), cut out toxic and chemically filled food, toxic chemical exposure, dairy, processed/junk/fried/fatty foods and cheap meats and other such irritants that are not going to contribute to the rebuilding of the gut. This is important because we do not want to cause more damage to the intestines at this point.

To further assist in the re-healing of the intestines we want to reduce stress. Stress can be in the form of chemical stress (addressed above), emotional stress in your day to day life and physical stress from injuries and harmful activities and habits.

Stress relates to the nervous system. When the body is stressed in one of these ways, the sympathetic nervous system switches on, this is the 'fight or flight' response, and straight away takes blood and energy away from the digestive system and puts it into the extremities to get the body ready to 'fight' or 'flight'.

By reducing stress we allow the body to revert back to the parasympathetic nervous system state, the 'rest and digest' state, and focus more on digestion and repair in the body. This is the state we need to be in.

Eat healthily. We want to predominantly consume fresh, organic, non-gmo and raw fruits and vegetables during the healing period. Blending these up will help at this point too for a better chance of assimilation into the body.

This is part of the attempt to heal the gut.

For more on this and a complete way to help heal the gut, please see the 'Leaky Gut' section of this book.

Cystic Fibrosis

What is it?

Cystic Fibrosis is a condition in which the epithelial cells (the protective layer of cells that line the organs and arteries) that secrete mucus produce a much thicker and stickier mucus because of a defective protein which clogs the bronchial tubes and thus interferes with breathing. It can also affect the digestive organs, such as the intestines and pancreas, and so the absorption of nutrients can be reduced leading to deficiencies and problems there also.

So, what causes it?

Most doctors will tell you that the problem comes down to genetics, but it has also been found that cystic fibrosis is caused by a deficiency in the essential trace mineral selenium.

Selenium is very important and essential for a wide range of functions within the body and you may have seen it mentioned in a few sections of this book for that very reason. It is important for the creation of many enzymes, one of which is the most powerful antioxidant in the body known as 'Glutathione Peroxidase' which helps to reduce the build-up of hydrogen peroxide and lipid hydro-peroxides which are fatty oxidised substances that decompose and form very harmful free radicals which are very dangerous that can and will attack any and everything they come into contact with including DNA. This can then cause mutations in the genes and lead to the complications we know as cystic fibrosis.

Symptoms

Symptoms can include persistent cough, problems gaining weight, difficulty breathing and shortness of breath, congested nasal and other respiratory symptoms such as lots of mucus building up in the sinuses, reoccurring pneumonia, fatigue, delay in physical growth and problems in the intestines (bloating and pale stools).

Solutions

As cystic fibrosis can and often does affect the gut of suffers, it is important to do what is possible to cleanse, heal and fortify the gut as having these gut issues can lead to a range of nutritional deficiencies which will then lead to a wide range of other problems in the body depending on the nutrient that becomes deficient.

For full info on how to go about doing this, please be sure to visit our 'Leaky Gut' section of this book.

So other than addressing the gut we must ensure that we have a sufficient amount of Selenium in the diet. This can be obtained from foods such as beans (lima), peas, nuts (brazil nuts and others), seeds (sunflower seeds, chia seeds, sesame seeds), mushrooms (like shiitake and button) and can be obtained in higher doses from supplemental form too.

Ensure to have sufficient intake of vitamin D (best source is the sun). In places where this is not possible, vitamin D supplements can be obtained and it is better to take Vitamin D3.

It is important to get sufficient amounts of Vitamin D into the system because cystic fibrosis can affect the pancreas and because of this there tends to be a problem with the breaking down of fat soluble vitamins such as A and E. Vitamin D can help keep the pancreas healthy amongst the wide range of other important roles it plays in the body.

To help reduce the mucus building up you should try to do things such as:

- Ensuring to consume lots of fresh and filtered water

- Doing some light exercise to stimulate the lymphatic system to help drain unwanted material out of the body

- Reduce your intake of mucus forming foods such as dairy, meats (especially cheap and/or fatty meats), sugar (and food that turns to sugar such as wheat, white rice, white potatoes and other starchy foods) and gluten (which is found in wheat, barley, rye and spelt).

Another great technique, which we also mention in the 'Asthma' section of this book, is to get a bowl of steaming hot water, put a few drops of tea tree oil into it, put a towel over the top of the bowl and your head and inhale slowly and deeply. Doing this until the steam disappears is a good way to break up the mucus a bit in the lungs which means you can then clear it out a lot easier.

If on medications, this will further deteriorate the gut lining. It is advisable then to do your best to move off of the drugs with the guidance of a healthcare professional. It is then possible to start taking measures that can help to heal this area. Again, for full information on this, see the 'Leaky Gut' section of this book.

As you will see mentioned in the 'Leaky Gut' section, food such as fresh, organic and raw fruits and vegetables are recommended, no processed foods or trans fats and you can help to stabilise the weight using natural foods and fats from things like avocados, olives, coconut, seeds, nuts and more.

Finally, boost the immune system to help the body fight off any infections and reduce the risk of pneumonia occurring or re-occurring. For detailed information on how to do this, see our 'Holistic Immune System Building' section.

By following these recommendations you should notice a marked difference in the condition.

Diabetes (Type 2)

What is it?
This condition is known as 'Insulin Resistance'. Type 1 diabetes is known as 'Insulin Dependent'. The majority of cases of people with diabetes are type 2.

Type 2 diabetes means the pancreas is under pressure to produce enough insulin for the amount of glucose present in the blood and/or that the cells are not able to take in the glucose that is present in the blood for whatever reason. As insulin is the factor that helps glucose enter a cell, we say the cells have become insulin resistant.

So, what causes it?
Genetics can make you more susceptible to getting diabetes, but as with most cases of genes playing a role in disease, it does not mean you will get it if you put in place the lifestyle changes that will help you to avoid it developing.

The predominant things that lead to diabetes are poor diet that is high in sugar, processed foods, artificial sweeteners and other chemicals and toxins, GMO foods, being overweight and inactivity.

Essentially this is a kind of lifestyle condition.

Symptoms
Symptoms of diabetes can be dry mouth and needing to drink regularly, increased hunger, increased urination, blurred vision, fatigue, slow healing from

cuts and wounds and tingling and/or numbness in hands or feet.

Solutions

As diabetes comes down to high blood sugar levels and a problem in the signalling that causes the insulin to essentially not open the door of the cell to let the glucose in, type 2 diabetes can be helped drastically by altering the diet.

It is especially important to be vigilant when trying to tackle this issue by committing to the changes. Changes would include things such as:

- Cutting out meats altogether for the healing period (especially fatty and cheap meats as most of these are fed on GMO feed and meat generally becomes acidic and can cause mucus in the body when digested)

- Cutting out dairy which is mucus forming

- Cutting out processed/junk and fried foods

- Eradicating the consumption of artificial sweeteners, colours, additives, preservatives and other toxins and synthetic chemicals that are present in foods and drinks

- Stopping alcohol consumption

- Stopping smoking

- Reducing or completely eliminating your intake

of things such as white potatoes, wheat (and other things made with wheat), grains such as white rice, pasta, bread, cereals, syrups, sweeteners and anything else that has a high glycemic index and turns to sugar in the system

- Work on losing weight if overweight

- Cut out refined and added sugars

With the system being cleared out in this way, we now want to give the body what it really needs.

This comes in the form of lots of fresh, organic and predominantly raw dark leafy green vegetables, other vegetables, low glycemic fruits such as lemons, limes, berries, grapefruit and watermelon (preferably in their whole state eaten as is or blended, not in concentrated or pre-bottled juices), nuts, seeds and good fats found in avocados, olives, coconuts and omega 3 fatty acids in fish oils, algae oils, seaweed such as wakame, ground chia seeds and flax seeds.

While this sounds somewhat restrictive, it is actually a very simple and highly effective way to re-establish good health in the body. It will help to reduce blood glucose levels naturally and bring back the insulin sensitivity of the cells as to reverse the insulin resistance and so it is one of the best ways to heal this condition.

Endometriosis

What is it?
This is a condition in females whereby the endometrial cells that line the inside of the uterus starts to grow in other places outside of the uterus, such as the bladder and ovaries.

So, what causes it?
Possible causes for this condition is too much oestrogen in the body, an impaired immune system which then makes getting rid of this excessive growth hard for the body and hormonal imbalances.

Symptoms
Symptoms can include pain in the pelvic area (especially around the time of menstruation) which could possibly increase with time, worse cramping than usual, pain when having sex, pain when urinating, excessive bleeding and infertility.

Solutions
Surgery for the condition is not always effective and it can still grow back after this so for this reason it is advisable to do things such as getting rid of toxins in the body from foods, water, external inputs and medications where possible (remember when ever thinking of coming off of a medication, do so with the supervision of a healthcare professional).

Some of these sources of toxins would be:

- Food – processed and junk foods because they contain a lot of synthetic ingredients and are predominantly nutrient deficient and cheap and/or fatty meats as they are fed on GMO feed which is proving to be very toxic and allergenic to the human organism

- Water – generally, tap water has been found to contain traces of lots of chemicals and heavy metals such as aluminium, arsenic, chlorine and others. For this reason you should always try and filter your water. The best kind of filters to get are 'Reverse Osmosis' filters or something like a 'Brita' filter

  It is also advisable to avoid bottled water that isn't in a 'BPA Free' plastic bottle as this is a toxic chemical that can actually leak into the water and then enter into the system

- External Inputs – other external inputs of toxins would include things like pollution from car fumes and other environmental toxins (which can't always be avoided, but try where possible) and chemicals used to clean and keep the home and body fresh (which all have natural alternatives)

- All medications contain toxic chemicals that cause harm to the body, this is why all medications have so many negative side effects

Eliminate foods such as:

- Dairy (as this is a mucus forming food)

- Wheat and foods with added sugar (fruits is the best way to get your sugars)

- Alcohol and caffeine which dehydrates the body and pulls out the essential nutrients it needs to function at full capacity and

- Soy which increases the oestrogen levels in the body and can make the condition worse

The best thing to do is to go fully organic, fresh and predominantly raw with fruit and vegetables during the healing period as this will help cleanse toxins out of the system and also reduce any excess acidity which will help the body keep in its slightly alkaline state.

Drink lots of fresh and filtered water and do your best to do some light exercise to help keep the lymphatic system stimulated and toxins flushing out of the body.

Another good idea is to do deep breathing as much as possible to help increase the levels of oxygen in the body.

Epilepsy

What is it?

Epilepsy is defined as reoccurring and spontaneous seizures. It is an electrical event in the body which is characterised by hyper excitability and hyper synchronicity of a large group of neurones at one time.

This essentially means that a surge of electricity in the body causes a part of the brain to fire many nerve cells at once causing a range of issues that are listed in the symptoms section below.

So, what causes it?

Some of the causes have been understood to be stress, infections, genetic susceptibility and can be alcohol induced when consumed in high amounts.

Symptoms

Depending on where the seizure takes place in the brain could mean varied symptoms, such as muscle twitching, unconsciousness, muscle stiffness, loss of muscle tone, sometimes the look of 'daydreaming' which they have a slight kind of black out and other such symptoms.

So it really depends on where in the brain the activity takes place.

Solutions

When we look at what epilepsy is and what has been found so far that could cause it, we must look at things that will help with the communication and signalling between the neurones as to not create a hyper excitable state in the system.

The first thing that comes to mind is neurotoxins.

Neurotoxins are known to interfere with the functioning and communication of the nerve cells in a range of ways. Essentially they are altering how the nerves act.

We know that today there are many neurotoxins around us. In the food (particularly processed and junk foods), water and medications. Have a look at the list below.

Some neurotoxins to be aware of are things like:

- Fluoride (which is found in many toothpastes, mouthwashes and water supplies)
- Pesticides, Herbicides and Fungicides (sprayed on literally all crops)
- MSG (Monosodium Glutamate - found in a wide range of foods - as a note, anything that says 'Flavouring' but is not defined as what exactly that is could very much be MSG)
- Aspartame and Sucralose (which are artificial sweeteners found in many foods and drinks - read ALL of your food labels - especially those things that say 'diet' and 'sugar free')
- Aluminium (found in vaccines, drinking water and medications)
- Mercury (which can be found in water, fish products, vaccines and tooth fillings).

So this should be the first thing to be aware of, neurotoxins and other chemicals that interfere with the natural functioning of our cells.

Things to avoid would be these toxins in the food, water, medications and car and industrial pollution but also the GMO food that is in circulation now.

Remember too that those animals that are not organically raised and grass fed are fed on GMO feed that then enters your body when you consume it. This includes the meat and milk from these animals.

Then we want to think of ways in which to strengthen the nervous system.

Strengthening the nervous system can be achieved by firstly strengthening the immune system as the two are linked. View the 'Holistic Immune System Building' section for more on this.

We can also strengthen the nervous system by ensuring that we are not giving excessive stress to the body in the form of toxins and chemicals as we addressed, but also medications, emotional stresses which comes from our everyday lives from worry, anxiety, being around negative people and having continuous negative thoughts and physical stresses in the form of injury and traumas to the body.

By reducing these stressors the body will not be in a heightened state all the time and more energy and time will be given to repairing and healing the body as opposed to gearing it up to 'fight' or 'flight'.

Vitamins obtained from foods and supplements can also help to keep the immune system and nervous system healthy, such as:

- Vitamin C which is very important as an antioxidant, in cellular function and hormone production

- Vitamin D which helps in the regulation of the development, function and protection of the nervous system and

- Selenium which is a precursor to one of the body's most powerful antioxidants and helps in the proliferation of white blood cells which protect the body. This coupled with:

- Vitamin E will make the effects even more powerful as Vitamin E also has great antioxidant effects and protects the nerve cells too which is going to help in keeping the nervous system strong and healthy.

Keeping the body moving is also going to be good (not too much, but just enough to stimulate the flow of blood and lymphatic system to help clean up excessive waste). Deep breathing to get efficient amounts of oxygen into the system to get to the cells, lots of fresh and filtered water, lots of fresh, organic fruits, vegetables, nuts, seeds and good fats which have a whole host of nutrients, minerals and the vitamins we mentioned.

Be sure to check out our 'Holistic Nervous System Building' section of the book for more information on keeping the nervous system healthy.

Eye Problems

What is it?
Any condition that affects the eyes. Here we shall focus on cataracts and glaucoma.

So, what causes it?
It is important to understand this: Most cells in the body need insulin in order to essentially open the cell door to allow glucose (sugar) in to be used as energy. There are some areas of the body that do not need to use insulin to get glucose to them, and this includes the eyes.

For this reason, many eye problems such as glaucoma and cataracts actually stem from a chronically high level of blood sugar which is why people with diabetes are at much higher risk of developing eye issues.

- Glaucoma is a condition of increased pressure in the eye that leads to gradual loss of sight

- Cataracts is a condition where the lens of the eye becomes increasingly blocked and thus vision is lost that way

Other causes in the case of Glaucoma can be from an increased pressure in the eye which can damage the optic nerve, having low blood pressure while having this increased eye pressure can actually restrict the needed blood flow to the eyes and lead to problem also.

Trauma and actual direct damage to the eyes can cause Glaucoma too. Chances can also be increased with family history of Glaucoma, increasing age and ethnicity such as African, Asian or Hispanic descent.

Other causes in the case of Cataract are due to just general ageing of the lens in the eyes, the use of some pharmaceutical drugs, nutritional deficiencies and even smoking and alcohol have been linked to this problem.

Symptoms
Symptoms can include blurred vision, loss of sight all together, bad vision at night, sensitivity to light, progressive sight worsening, colours fading and double vision in one eye.

Solutions
One of the main solutions to eye problems in general is to ensure you reduce your sugar intake as this can directly affect the eyes. It is also important to reduce intake of chemicals that can get into the blood stream and make the system toxic.

Then with these in check, it is advisable to eat foods that have all of the nutrients and minerals your body needs to repair, grow and stay strong and healthy which can be found in fresh, organic and predominantly raw vegetables (lots of dark leafy greens too), low glycemic fruits such as lemons, limes, watermelon and berries, nuts, seeds, mushrooms and good fats such as avocado, olives, coconut, fish oils, algae oils, seaweed such as wakame, ground chia seeds and flax seeds.

More specific to the eyes, as you probably know, Vitamin A is good for eye health so anything that contains 'beta-carotene', which turns to Vitamin A in the body, will be beneficial here and this is most foods that are orange and yellow in colour such as carrots, peppers, squash and the like.

Finally, it is important to have a good intake of zinc for eye health as this protects and reduces aging of the eyes.

Keep these kind of solutions going to help your body do what it does best, and that is to heal and sustain itself.

Fibromyalgia

What is it?
Characterised as an auto immune disease, fibromyalgia is literally a condition by which everything aches and hurts, the person feels constant fatigue, tenderness and other such problems.

So, what causes it?
When we look at the symptoms you will see some similarities between this condition and the symptoms of 'Celiacs disease'. Also it may be important to mention here that they are both considered as auto immune diseases which essentially means the body is attacking itself.

Celiac is a problem in the gut and most auto immune diseases actually start in the gut too. When the 'villi' (hair like extensions that line the intestinal walls) are damaged and the walls of the intestinal tract becomes compromised and spaces form, undigested proteins that are in the intestines can pass through the walls and enter the blood stream.

This is not supposed to happen, only amino acids are used by the body by getting absorbed through the villi and for this reason proteins have to be broken down properly by the stomach for this assimilation to be successful.

When these proteins get into the blood stream, the body sees them as invaders and mounts an attack against them. Antibodies are then formed to attack this whenever they see it.

Something then happens called 'molecular mimicry' in which the antibodies start to identify other proteins in the body as the invader and attack them too. This is because there are thousands of different combinations of proteins in the body acting out different roles such as enzyme creation and producing connective tissues etc so the likeliness of an undigested protein looking like one of your own proteins is quite high which is why this happens.

This can happen with any organ or tissue in the body as they all use proteins and this is what we call an auto immune disease.

Symptoms
Pain all over the body, tenderness, joint problems, fatigue, depression and other such symptoms.

Solutions
The solution to this problem is to ensure that first and foremost the GI tract is healthy. This includes ensuring that the stomach has the right concentration of stomach acid so it can break down the proteins and then ensuring that the small intestine is not damaged so that it can do its job and absorb only the broken down proteins, fats and carbohydrates.

For full info on these two elements see the 'Acid Reflux' section of this book (with regards to stomach acid) and the 'Leaky Gut' section of this book.

Next we want to essentially help calm down and desensitise the system, give the body all of the nutrients, vitamins and minerals it needs and, as best we can, just help the body to do what it does best, and that is heal itself.

So once we know how to best try and heal the GI tract from the stomach down, we want to ensure the body is out of a stressed state in terms of chemical stress which can come from toxins and chemicals in food, water, pollution, products we use for washing our clothes, house and body and medications. We also have to be aware of emotional stress which comes from our everyday life in the way we view the world around us, interact with people, think about the situations in our life and choose the people we regularly spend time with. Finally we must be aware of physical stress from injuries and traumas we inflict on our bodies, both internally and externally.

When our body is in a stressful state, it takes away the supply of blood and energy from the digestive system and instead uses that for the 'fight' or 'flight' response type of action.

These are known as the parasympathetic (rest and digest) and sympathetic (fight or flight) nervous system states. It is also interesting to note that when the gut is damaged, brain function can be affected too which is why, along with the fact of being in constant pain, depression can develop in people with fibromyalgia.

We want to do what we can to let the body heal itself in the parasympathetic state.

At the same time, you want to ensure you have a

good functioning nervous system so it can work to its maximum capability whilst in this state which will include ensuring you have good posture, getting sufficient deep sleep and rest, light exercise (just to your ability - as this will also stimulate the lymphatic system), deep breathing as much as often and meditation should be considered too.

Please also be sure to check out our 'Holistic Nervous System Building' section of this book and the 'Holistic Immune System Building' section for further detailed information.

Gallstones

What is it?
This is a condition whereby crystals form in the gallbladder due to too much cholesterol compared to bile acid being secreted by the liver and gallbladder.

When this happens, the cholesterol does not get dissolved fully and forms into these crystals which can block the bile ducts and cause a lot of pain and problems.

It is when the system is blocked up like this, that infection can form in the ducts which can then spread into the blood stream and then to other parts of the body.

So, what causes it?
Being overweight can be a cause here, as excessive cholesterol can be present in the body in an overweight person.

A diet high in fatty food, sugar, toxic and chemically laden foods such as processed foods and junk foods can also be a cause here as this can also cause a higher cholesterol production compared to bile. These things can also lead to 'fatty liver' which is essentially fat build-ups in the liver and thus the bile creation and secretion is decreased too. It is the liver that secretes the bile and stores it in the gallbladder.

We must also remember that cholesterol is a precursor to stress hormones such as cortisol which are reactions to the body being in a stressed state. So when the body is physically, chemically or emotionally stressed, more cholesterol will be produced.

Medications that alter the liver enzymes can also cause issues and medications such as birth control and hormone pills because high levels of oestrogen can decrease the contraction of the gall bladder and also makes the bile thicker which can then lead to the development of the gallstones. This is why women are more susceptible to gallstones than men because women generally have higher levels of oestrogen in the body.

Something else that affects the liver that can also contribute to gallstones is hepatitis, which is inflammation of the liver.

Symptoms

Symptoms can include constant abdominal pain, pain in the back on the right side, sharp pains, problems breathing deeply and pain after eating meals.

Solutions

First and foremost, try not to get the gallbladder removed if you are suffering from this (unless you absolutely have too in severe cases) as this can really stop you from digesting fats properly and absorbing nutrients further down in the intestines. This is because bile is used to help break up the fats you eat and stop the food you eat being too acidic as it travels further down through the digestive system.

- Try to control your diet by eating less fatty,

greasy, processed, fried and junk foods to avoid this excessive build-up of cholesterol.

- Reduce alcohol, fizzy drinks and caffeine as these will dehydrate your body and could lead to the bile becoming thicker. Drink lots of fresh and filtered water.

- Eat good amounts of turmeric which will help stop gallstones forming.

- Ensure to have good levels of Vitamin C and D and reduce your levels of sugar intake.

To dissolve the larger gallstones you can try things such as drinking lots of fresh lemons squeezed into water regularly and try drinking a few drops of apple cider vinegar mixed in water.

Gout

What is it?

This condition is a type of arthritis in which there is too much uric acid in the body which then forms into crystals in the joints, especially the toes. Men are much more susceptible to Gout than women.

So, what causes it?

As old muscle and tissue cells break down in the body (known as purines) they do so into uric acid. This happens on a daily basis.

Things such as meats, alcohol and sugary drinks and foods will increase the amount of uric acid in the body. Generally we get rid of this excessive uric acid through the kidneys, but if the kidneys are not functioning properly, even more uric acid will be present.

With age, the kidneys get less and less efficient and at the same time the body begins to break down faster. So this will cause the build-up of the uric acid but if you also have a problem with your kidneys, it will happen much faster.

Dehydration is also a cause leading to the condition and previous illnesses that may have further deteriorated the body and slowed down kidney function. Caffeine poses a problem here with regards to dehydration because caffeine affects the kidneys by stimulating them to release too much water from the body.

There are also foods that can be eaten that will increase the amount of uric acid, these include: sea food, meat, beans, mushrooms and high fructose corn syrup and other refined sugars (found in lots of fast and junk foods).

Other causes can include:

- Medications that alter the functioning of the kidneys or that are toxic to the system, thereby increasing the load the kidneys have to filter from the blood, and

- Hypothyroidism which slows the metabolism of all processes in the body which can then lead to more uric acid being stored instead of disposed of

Symptoms
Possible symptoms of Gout can include pain in the joints, especially the feet and toes, swelling and tenderness.

Solutions
To try and break down the uric acid in the body a few things should be considered, such as eating lots of celery and drinking celery juice, black cherries, nettles and lots of fresh and filtered water will help to flush the body and reduce the amount of uric acid build up.

Things to avoid to help lower the continuous levels of uric acid in the body should be things such as alcohol, sugars (and things that break down into sugar such as lots of grains and starchy foods), caffeine and meats.

If possible, reduce or cut out the medications that you take but remember to always do this with the supervision of a healthcare professional.

Take processed and junk foods, artificial sweeteners and other synthetic chemicals out of your diet as these will make the blood more acidic. It is when the blood is in a more acidic state that problems start to occur. So keeping the body in its naturally slightly alkaline state will be the best thing to do when trying to heal and detox the body.

Ionised water is a good idea to be used but you have to ensure that the water source you use is fresh, clean water not full of chemicals otherwise chemicals will be concentrated when you ionise the water.

This works because when you put something very alkaline in the stomach the acid in the stomach has a longer way to go to get down to a low acidic state, which is where the stomach likes to be. This is good because for every molecule of hydrochloric acid secreted into the stomach a molecule of sodium bicarbonate is secreted into the blood which alkalises the system.

When the blood is too acidic and not enough sodium bicarbonate is produced, the body starts to leech calcium from the bones in order to alkalise the blood which can lead to other problems such as osteoporosis.

This is not something you should drink all of the time,

but can be very affective during the healing period.

Eat foods that will help the body stay in its slightly alkaline state, such as lots of fresh, organic and raw fruit and vegetables as much as possible which also gives the body a wide range of nutrients and vitamins which promotes good health.

Gum Disease

What is it?
Gum disease is caused by the build-up of plaque because of a large amount of bacteria being present in the mouth. As this bacteria build up worsens and is left unchecked, tooth decay and gum disease starts to occur, such as gingivitis (inflamed gums) and periodontitis (damage to the soft tissue and bone that supports the teeth).

So, what causes it?
This condition is caused by a build-up of bacteria in the mouth predominantly from the residues of food and drink which have not been properly removed. The bacteria is then given the opportunity to multiply and grow and the problems we know to be tooth decay and gum disease then become known.

Symptoms
Symptoms can include constant bad breath, bleeding gums, swollen and tender gums, loose teeth, loss of teeth and pain when chewing and eating.

Solutions
It is important to keep gum health in check because when disease starts to set in, the bacteria present can start to spread to other parts of the body which will cause further disease and issues in other areas so also keep on top of tooth and oral health.

Some really great solutions for gum disease and general oral health are things such as:

'Oil pulling' - this is where you put some oil into your mouth and swish it around and pull it back and forth through your teeth for around 15 – 20 minutes ensuring you cover all areas of the mouth and then spit it out. The best oils for this are sesame seed oil and coconut oil. Doing this has really great anti-bacterial effects and the nutrients in the oils help to keep the teeth and gums strong and healthy.

Gargling with salt is also very anti-bacterial and will keep an excess bacteria build up at bay.

Neem is another great thing you can use to keep your teeth and gums healthy, which is a bark that you can get in natural toothpastes and as a powder.

A paste of turmeric root, rock salt and mustard seed oil can be rubbed into the gums and left for a few minutes before washing your mouth out as a method to increase tooth and gum health.

If your gum disease has got very bad, a very powerful solution called white oak bark powder can be used and is very effective in re-strengthening the teeth, gums and surrounding areas in the mouth.

General everyday things to do to reduce gum diseases and increase oral health includes such things as reducing the amount of sugary foods, processed foods and junk foods and drinks you consume, brush properly and regularly, drink fresh and filtered water, eat organic and fresh fruits and vegetables but remember fruit contains sugar too so ensure to always brush regularly and properly.

Doing these things should help you keep your oral hygiene up to a very high standard and get rid of excessive bacterial growth and gum disease.

While it is common for dentists to suggest fluoride it really should be avoided in every possible way. While fluoride may harden the enamel of the teeth, in excess it can actually cause the opposite effect and produce a condition called 'Fluorosis', but much more importantly fluoride has been shown to be a neurotoxin and is very detrimental to the rest of the body and accumulates in the system affecting the nervous system and endocrine system. Fluoride should be avoided at all costs.

Hayfever

What is it?

Hayfever is an allergy based condition, whereby the immune system becomes hyperactive and hyper responsive and reacts to harmless things such as pollen. The body then releases histamine to combat these 'intruders' which cause the symptoms associated with Hayfever.

So, what causes it?

There are a few things that can cause the immune system to become hyperactive and hyper responsive, and these are things such as chemicals in the body, sugar, vaccines (which again are full of chemicals) and other neurotoxins.

Some neurotoxins to be aware of are things like:

- Fluoride (which is found in many toothpastes, mouthwashes and water supplies)
- Pesticides (sprayed on crops)
- Herbicides and Fungicides (sprayed on crops)
- MSG (Monosodium Glutamate - found in a wide range of foods - as a note, anything that says 'Flavouring' could very much be MSG)
- Aspartame and Sucralose (which are artificial sweeteners found in many foods and drinks - read ALL of your food labels - especially those things that say 'diet' and 'sugar free')
- Aluminium (found in vaccines, drinking water and medications)
- Mercury (which can be found in water, fish products, vaccines and tooth fillings).

What these chemicals do is essentially alter the way the neurones and cells communicate with each other, compromise immune function and thus alter the way in which the body reacts to outside stimuli.

Symptoms

Symptoms can include sneezing, running nose, watering eyes, itchy eyes and nose, heaviness in head and itchy throat.

Solutions

There are a few things that can help reduce the symptoms, build immunity and detox the body of chemicals. Those that reduce symptoms and build immunity are:

Nettles, vitamin c, grapes and grape seed extract, fresh organic fruit (like pineapple, oranges, cranberries and blueberries) and lots of vegetable juices and blends with dark leafy greens.

As this is an allergic reaction, see the 'Leaky Gut' page to see how the gut can relate to allergies and how to go about correcting this aspect of it, if it stems from this. If you have a range of other allergies or intolerances to food, it could well be from a leaky gut.

Avoid GMOS, processed foods, junk foods, artificial sweeteners and other such chemicals like pesticides etc to help the body move out of a stressed state, in this case chemical stress. By doing this it will help the body move into a state where it can calm down and heal.

It is also advisable to get a good amount of exercise and avoid drinking alcohol and smoking.

You can reduce the mucus and cleanse the sinuses by using a 'Neti Pot' which is a pot that allows you to put slightly salty water up one nostril and let it run through the sinuses and out of the other nostril and the repeat on the other side which helps to flush out mucus and congestion in this area.

The other method is to get a bowl of streaming hot water, put a few drops of tea tree oil in it and put a towel over your head and the bowl. Inhale the vapours for as long as the water is steaming and this will help to cleanse the sinuses too.

By cleansing the body and doing things that help to relax the nervous system, you can notice a great difference in hayfever symptoms.

Hepatitis (A-E)

What is it?

Hepatitis refers to the inflammation of the liver. The different types of Hepatitis (A, B, C, D and E) refers to the virus causing the hepatitis and can indicate how it was contracted too.

Hepatitis A and E are very similar, in that they are the less damaging kind and generally people can get past these kinds of hepatitis. They are known as the 'environmental' kind as you can contract them from things such as contaminated water/food/faeces and through unprotected sex with a contaminated person.

Hepatitis B, C and D on the other hand are the more damaging kind. Hepatitis B and D are very similar to each other and you actually need to have Hepatitis B in order to even get D. These two are generally contracted through things such as needle sharing with someone who has got it (IV), through sex and passed from mother to child during birth. C is also very similar and in the past it was known to be passed sometimes in blood transfusions.

The virus enters the liver cells and starts to replicate itself, which triggers the immune cells to come and attack, causing inflammation and death of the cells. This then leads to scaring of those areas and inhibits the liver from doing its job properly (this scarring is known as 'Cirrhosis' which shortens the flow of blood in and out of the liver and shrinks and hardens the liver).

So, what causes it?

Hepatitis is a lot of the time caused by one the viruses mentioned above, which is why they have a letter to say what kind of virus it is. So people generally contract it by being exposed to the virus from the above mentioned means.

There is another way of getting hepatitis, or inflammation of the liver, and that is through chronic alcohol use. This is known as 'alcoholic hepatitis'.

Symptoms

Symptoms can include jaundice (yellowish skin, eyes and fingernails), dark urine, light coloured stools, nausea, fatigue, fever, abdominal pain, poor appetite and 'flu like' symptoms.

Solutions

So what can we do about Hepatitis?

Some of the main overarching things that need to be considered is to:

- **Vitalise the body and resolve toxins in the system**
  You can do this with things such as fresh, organic and raw fruits and vegetables that contain lots of minerals, nutrients, vitamins and enzymes that will clear the body of toxins and boost the overall health of the system.

If you have been reading this book all the way through so far, you may find a lot of these things repetitive, but that is because the body is a self-regulating system and if given the correct environment internally will do what it does best and that is heal itself.

- Flush the liver and reduce phlegm in the body
We can do this by taking things such as dandelion root, garlic, milk thistle, beetroot, lemon water and lots of dark leafy greens.

These things will also help to cleanse the blood too.

If the kidneys are not functioning to their full potential this can worsen the condition so ensure to boost and strengthen the kidneys by ensuring your diet is not too high in protein (still adequate amounts though), reduce the toxins and chemicals you introduce into the body and stay hydrated.

Nourish and cleanse the blood and ensure there are no stagnations in the system anywhere which can be done through keeping the body moving (some exercise) and eating foods that help to cleanse the bloodstream as mentioned above.

Ensure to have sufficient amounts of Selenium, Vitamin D, Vitamin C and Vitamin E in the body as these are extremely important in the development, health and protection of the body, so having good amounts of these will help strengthen immune cells, detox the body and slow the spread of the virus a little more.

Other foods to include would be things like Chlorella, rhubarb root, turmeric, garlic, onions, broccoli and red peppers.

Finally, using the advice above will also strengthen and keep the spleen healthy which is important as the spleen and liver are closely related.

High Cholesterol

What is it?
High cholesterol is the high accumulation of cholesterol fat in the blood. It is not a disease in and of itself, but a reaction to something else happening in the body.

Cholesterol is actually very important for the creation and maintenance of every cell in the body as it helps the cells to communicate and forms every single cells membrane.

It is important for the creation of the bile salts. Bile salts help to break down the fats that we eat and release the fat soluble vitamins A, D, E and K to allow them to be absorbed in the intestines. It is also a precursor to our steroidal hormones such as testosterone, oestrogen and progesterone and stress hormones such as Cortisol. So as you can see, it is very important.

You may have heard of 'good' cholesterol and 'bad' cholesterol. Whilst those terms may not be exactly how to class them, there are differences between the two.

It may make more sense if we explain it:

When you have high cholesterol you have a high amount of lipids in your blood, in this case fats. Lipids come in two types, triglycerides and cholesterol. We have mentioned what cholesterol does and triglycerides are used for energy from the food you eat.

In the liver, lipids are wrapped in proteins that allow them to travel through the body, this is called a 'lipoprotein' and depending on what lipoprotein the cholesterol is wrapped in, will determine the type of cholesterol that travels around the body.

The liver produces a lot of LDL cholesterol (known as the 'bad' cholesterol) when the body is under some form of stress whether chemical, emotional or physical and is used for repair. It can build up in the blood and create plaques that stick to and cause damage to blood vessels when prolonged. This will then narrow the passage of the blood vessels, restrict the blood flow and make the blood pressure increase in order to still get blood to everywhere it is needed.

On the other hand, the liver creates HDL cholesterol too. This helps to remove the excessive build-up of cholesterol from the body and arteries and takes it back to the liver (which is why it is called the 'good' cholesterol).

So, what causes it?
The build-up of LDL cholesterol can happen due to stresses on the body as we have mentioned, which triggers the release of the cholesterol to essentially go and fix some kind of problem in the body and allows the stress hormones to be activated. This can be triggered by foods high in fats, chemicals and artificial substances, refined carbohydrates, alcohol, sugar, fast food and junk foods (which are all chemical stressors), but also by emotional worries and physical problems too.

When LDL predominates over HDL this is where the build-up can continue and problems start to occur in the system.

Symptoms

There are generally not many symptoms to high cholesterol except from sometimes noticing high blood pressure and related reactions.

Solutions

So how can we manage the balance of LDL and HDL cholesterol?

There are a range of things we can do to naturally control cholesterol, and these are:

First and foremost, get the body out of a stressed state. We can get the body out of a stressed state by reducing chemical, emotional and physical stresses on the body to allow the system to return to the parasympathetic state which is the 'rest and digest' state of the nervous system.

We also want to ensure to:

- Have regular exercise and lose any excess weight as this is vital to helping the body heal itself and return to a healthy state. Carrying excessive weight and not doing much physical exercise will not help in rectifying the situation

- Eat healthier fats from foods such as

avocados, olives, nuts, seeds and coconut (and yes you do need saturated fats in your diet, but that doesn't mean too much of it - you can get this from coconuts and as a bonus you get the rejuvenating properties of them too)

- Avoid trans fats and hydrogenated oils

- Avoid artificial sweeteners, colours and flavourings

- Stop smoking and drinking

- Eat as much organic, fresh and raw foods as possible which will help to revitalise, heal and strengthen the body, include nuts and seeds in here too

- Try your best to come off of statins (cholesterol lowering medications) because, as we mentioned, you need cholesterol, you just need to make some changes to ensure your ratio of LDL to HDL is good

  Drugs will not help you do this and will cause further chemical stresses to your body and will inhibit enzymes in your liver which over time will cause damage to the organ

- Increase Omega-3 fatty acid intake. Good sources of this are fish and fish oils, algae oils, hemp seeds, ground flax seeds and chia seeds and seaweed like wakame

High cholesterol can very easily be rectified by understanding what the body needs and then implementing those changes to produce the ideal environment for healing to take place and vitality to be restored.

Hives

What is it?
Hives is an allergy based reaction to a few different things such as different foods, medications, certain chemicals and other such things which can vary from person to person. This can be a chronic condition or can be severe as to be anaphylactic.

It is like a rash that comes and goes. It can come up one place, go down and then come up somewhere else.

So, what causes it?
We can look at this from two angles here. The first is the fact that it is a skin condition. Many skin conditions indicate that there are toxins in the blood that are trying to be excreted through the nearest port, that being the skin.

Secondly, it is an allergic reaction that can come from foods and other means. For that reason we must look at the gut as the gut is very much involved in allergic reactions in many cases. For more details on the gut and allergy connection, see our 'Leaky Gut' section of the book.

Whatever the cause may be, the body has become hyper-sensitive to the allergen.

Symptoms
Symptoms can include swollen skin, rashes, itchiness

and slight pain for some people.

Solutions

So as this is a skin related condition, we must treat the body for toxins and toxic chemicals.

For this we can detox the body with things such as regular exercise, reducing stress in the form of chemical, emotional and physical stressors on the body as this puts the body into the sympathetic nervous system state (the 'fight' or 'flight' state) which alters how the digestive system works and keeps the body in a unrelaxed state.

You would have probably read this in the 'Holistic Nervous System Building' section, but here are some causes of the different stressed states:

-   Chemical stresses: medications, vaccines, pollution from cars and industrial fumes, chemicals and heavy metals in the water supply and synthetic chemicals in the food we eat which are predominantly in processed, junk and fast foods but also sprayed on all crops. Also be aware of the 'nightshades' group of foods which can cause problems in the gut and cause permeability which then allows toxins to leak into the blood stream. Nightshades consist of tomatoes, tobacco, potatoes, egg-plant and peppers

-   Emotional stresses: From negative thoughts, worrying about situations, anxiety, depression, being around unsupportive and negative people, having a pessimistic view of the world and situations and other such stressful things

- Physical stresses: From injuries, wounds, burns, pain, strains and other related physical pressures

Next, as this can also be allergy based, we want to address and heal the gut as there will probably be some issues here too. For a full, detailed plan on how to heal the gut which will also help the body to detox itself and absorb the nutrients that are needed for the healthy rebuilding of cells, please refer to our 'Leaky Gut' section.

On this page you will also get a full list of the best foods to utilise when going about healing the body and moving away from such a condition.

Hyperglycaemia

What is it?
High blood sugar is just that, when the sugar levels in the blood are too high for the system and thus puts a strain on the circulatory system and causes damage to the arteries and other organs.

High blood sugar, just like high cholesterol, is not a disease in and of itself, but an indicator that something else is going on in the body.

So, what causes it?
Hyperglycaemia can be caused by a range of things such as a high intake of sugary foods (or foods that turn into sugar such as grains like wheat, starchy foods, processed foods and junk foods) that will then build up in the blood stream. This can worsen when there is lack of exercise too as it will build up quicker in a body that is stagnant.

Another reason is a lack of insulin being able to open the cells to get the glucose in where it is needed (such as in diabetes). For more on this concept please visit our 'Diabetes (Type 2)' section.

Other reasons include the body being in a stressed state, either chemically, physically and/or emotionally. This then releases stress hormones that raise the blood sugar and blood pressure in an attempt to prepare the body for a fight or flight response. The body then stays in this state if not addressed and the problem persists.

Finally, hyperglycaemia can be caused by bacteria, viruses and other illnesses as this too is a stressor on the body.

Symptoms

Symptoms can include dry mouth, lethargy, blurred vision, dry skin, feeling sick, tired/drowsiness, increased infection rate and finally:

The "3 Poly's" which are:
- Polydipsia (drinking a lot of fluids)
- Polyuria (going to the toilet much more than usual) and
- Polyphagia (excessive hunger due to glucose not getting into the cells where it is needed which makes you hungry because your cells are literally being starved of energy)

It is important to note that there are certain cells in the body that do not need insulin in order to get their energy. One of these is the eyes as we mentioned in the diabetes section of the book and because of this they can become easily damaged with chronic states of Hyperglycaemia.

Solutions

The solutions to Hyperglycaemia are the same solutions as the 'Diabetes (Type 2)' solutions, so please visit that section in this book.

This will mainly focus on the insulin and high blood sugar relationship, but remember to also address the stressed state of the body to relax it back into the parasympathetic state and thus allow the body to return to a state that is conducive to healing.

Hypoglycaemia

What is it?
Hypoglycaemia is the opposite of hyperglycaemia.
This is low blood sugar.

So, what causes it?
Low blood sugar is most often found in diabetics.
While that sounds paradoxical as diabetes is about
high blood sugar, diabetics can sometimes take too
much insulin and other blood glucose reducing
medications and thus their blood sugar can drastically
drop or because they are on insulin if they do not eat
enough, their glucose levels will again drop to low
amounts in the blood.

For people who do not have diabetes, low blood
sugar can come from being on certain medications,
thyroid problems, alcohol abuse or diseases of the
stomach, kidney, liver or pancreas. So it is advisable
to get all of these checked.

All of these can lead to the body not being able to
convert food into glucose properly and store it in the
body for later use.

Chronic low blood sugar is less common than chronic
high blood sugar, although for diabetics it is seen very
often.

Symptoms
Symptoms can include Irritability, confusion, fast
heartbeat, light headedness, blurred vision, tingling or

numbness in the lips or tongue, hunger, nausea, tiredness, shakiness, anxiety, sweating, chills and clamminess.

Solutions

For many people, the way to get their blood sugar back to good levels is to just eat something that is easily converted to sugar in order to get it into the blood quickly.

For those without diabetes and who have continual low blood sugar, it is important to get the thyroid, stomach, kidneys, liver and pancreas checked and reduce the amount of alcohol consumption if that is something that is an issue. Another thing would be to have a look at any medications being taken to see if these are the cause of the problem.

For those with diabetes, which is the majority cases of hypoglycaemia, it is important to ensure that the intake of food is sufficient in relation to the amount of insulin being taken. Hypothyroid can also play a role in patients with diabetes.

This insulin to food intake ratio may have to be monitored and in certain circumstances adjusted with the help of a healthcare professional to ensure it is not unnecessarily putting the person into a low blood sugar state often, as this can be very dangerous as all cells in the body need glucose for energy to function correctly.

Another thing to consider is that if the person has started to heal themselves of type 2 diabetes (see our

'Diabetes (Type 2)' page for more info on that), their insulin sensitivity of the cells can start to increase again which means external insulin taken will again have to be lowered to not cause the hypoglycaemic state.

Hypertension

What is it?
As with high blood sugar, high blood pressure is not a disease in and of itself either. It is an indicator that something else is happening in the body that is forcing the heart to work harder in order to keep the blood flowing to all of the cells and tissues.

Generally, someone should not just start taking high blood pressure medications without first seeking out the cause of the high blood pressure. Otherwise this can just cause the body to be put under further stress while it tries to keep everything running.

In chronic and prolonged cases, hypertension will actually wear down the heart muscle and the arteries and increase the risk of heart disease, heart attacks and strokes.

Of course in emergency cases, someone may need to take the medication to avoid heart attacks and such.

So, what causes it?
When the body receives chemical, emotional and/or physical stress, the blood pressure naturally rises to give more energy to the extremities to be ready for a flight or fight response (this is the sympathetic nervous system).

Blood sugar levels will also be raised during this time due to the stress hormones that are released, such as cortisol, which aim to increase the levels of the sugar and blood to ensure you have enough energy to respond to any perceived threat.

All medications cause a chemical stress to the body, which if continuously taken over long periods of time will keep the body in a chemically stressed state, thereby in many cases ensuring that these levels will always be raised. This will also affect the functioning of the liver and kidneys as the medications make the blood toxic which has to be filtered predominantly through the kidneys but also the liver.

If overweight, and especially if the body is in an inactive state a lot of the time, the heart has to work harder to pump blood around the system. If this is unnaturally suppressed, whether it reads well on a test or not, this will not be helping your system to regulate and keep itself running and will cause damage in the long term.

Smoking, drinking alcohol, eating lots of chemically filled and high fatty and sugary foods (and foods that turn to sugar) and all types of stress will contribute to raising your blood pressure levels. These will dehydrate the body too which will make the blood thicker and the pressure rise.

Symptoms
Symptoms can include headaches, chest pain, vision problems, difficulty in breathing, irregular heartbeat, thumping in head, neck and/or chest.

Solutions
When checking your blood pressure, you should not

just check it once and take that as your proper blood pressure reading. You should check it around 3 times a day. One in the morning, one at midday and one at night over a few days period to get an average reading. You should do one laying down, one sitting and one standing up. This will give you a much more accurate and reliable reading of what your normal blood pressure is and what it is really doing.

You want to get good deep sleep and rest, lots of hydration with fresh and filtered water and de-stress yourself in all ways (physically, emotionally and chemically) and do light exercise to help keep the blood flowing, the lymphatic system removing excessive toxins and the body pushing them out through sweat.

Getting out in the sun regularly, visiting the beach and natural environments is also a very good way to de-stress, get lots of fresh oxygen and get some light exercise all in one scoop. Whilst doing this do deep breathing as much as you can from the diaphragm.

As is always advised through-out this book, and for good reason, it is going to be a big part of this solution that you eat lots of fresh, organic and predominantly raw fruits and vegetables to help detox the body, get the sufficient amount of minerals, vitamins and nutrients needed and keep the body strong and vibrant.

Your diet should consist of fruits, vegetables, nuts, seeds and good fats (these good fats are found in avocados, olives, coconut oil (for your healthy source of saturated fat that the cells need), fish oils, algae oils, flax and chia seeds and seaweed such as wakame (for your essential omega 3 fatty acids) and you will also get your good fats from the nuts and seeds too.

Specific foods to consume which will be beneficial would be things like eating celery, garlic, onions, oregano, basil, fennel and hemp seeds.

- Getting out in the sun regularly for Vitamin D is also advisable

- Meditate as much as you can to calm the mind and body which will help in moving the nervous system out of the stressed, sympathetic state

Things to probably avoid are:

- Dairy (for calcium eat lots of dark leafy greens)

- Canned foods

- Fatty Meats

- Table salt and salts added to food (use small amounts of sea salt)

- Reduce or stop alcohol intake

- Reduce and come off of medications (do this with the supervision of a healthcare professional)

- Reduce sugar intake (and foods that turn to sugar like grains, breads, pastas, other starchy foods and refined sugars such as corn starch and high fructose corn syrup found in processed foods)

- Processed and junk foods

Remember, hypertension is an indicator that something else is happening in the body. It is advisable to try the suggestions above before considering taking any medications for the condition.

Hypotension

What is it?
Just like hypertension, hypotension is not a disease in itself either but again an indicator that something else is happening in the body. There can be a range of causes for low blood pressure and many people can have low blood pressure without realising it as having low blood pressure is not generally a dangerous thing unless of course it becomes too low and symptoms are then starting to be experienced.

So, what causes it?
There are a range of causes for hypotension, one of the most common causes is low blood volume which can be caused by a haemorrhage, loss of fluids from not drinking enough water (dehydration), vomiting and diarrhoea. Low blood volume can also come about from excessive sweating, large burns and diuretics too.

Other causes of low blood pressure are widening of the blood vessels, hormonal changes, medication side effects such as beta blockers and anti-depressants, heart problems and also endocrine problems. Then there is also the inability to retain electrolytes, heart conditions and finally a problem with the autonomic nervous system which regulates blood pressure.

So there are a wide range of causes for it.

Symptoms

Symptoms can include dizziness/light headed (especially when going from sitting to standing), fainting, weakness in limbs, chest pain, consistent dehydration, going into shock, coldness, blurred vision and blue nails and tongue.

Solutions

We must first remember that having low blood pressure is not always a bad thing. It can actually be very healthy as long as it doesn't fall too low.

In the cases where it does fall too low, there are a few things that should be kept in mind, such as:

-   Ensuring you have a sufficient intake of fresh and filtered water to avoid dehydration which is one of the causes of low blood volume that can lead to low blood pressure. As the kidneys also have a significant role to play in water and mineral retention, it will be important to get them checked too

-   If you are on any medications it is important to check to see if these medications are causing the issues. Have a look at the side effects and possible reactions they can cause. It would be advisable to do what you can to come off any medications you are taking as these add toxicity to the body and can put more tax on the organs. Remember to always do this with the assistance of a healthcare professional to be safe though.

-   Breathing exercises such as 'Pranayama'

which can have two benefits for those with hypotension. One is that certain techniques can increase the heat in the body and help to raise the blood pressure naturally and one such Pranayama breathing technique is called 'Bhastrika' and the other benefit is that it can help relax and realign the autonomic nervous system which controls the blood pressure

- Cut down on alcohol consumption and smoking as these can add toxicity to the system which affects the blood pressure amongst other things

- Reduce caffeine intake which acts as a diuretic

- Have adequate amounts of sea salt. Salt is actually used and needed by the body (as it is sodium and chloride). The problem comes when we have too much salt and especially generic table salt. So it is advisable to get small amounts of sea salt. Sea salt is better because it hasn't been stripped of the natural minerals that are present there whereas table salt has.

Remember if a person has low blood pressure without any of the signs and the symptoms we discussed, it should be ok as having healthy low blood pressure is a good thing.

If someone has a bad case of it, it is advisable to get the liver, kidneys and heart checked for any problems there.

Hyperthyroid

What is it?
The thyroid controls the metabolism of all of the processes in the body (how quickly or slowly all processes happen in the body). In this condition where the thyroid is overactive, things will be happening in the body too fast and as a result problems can occur such as the things detailed in the symptoms section.

So, what causes it?
This condition is much less common when compared to 'hypothyroidism' (explained next), but some of the most common causes for this condition are factors such as 'Grave's Disease' which is classed as an auto immune disease where the TSH (Thyroid Stimulating Hormone) is mimicked and produces too much which then causes the thyroid to produce too much of its hormones T3 and T4 which is used in the body for control of the metabolism. So Grave's Disease is the most common cause for the condition.

If it is not down to Grave's Disease, other things that can lead to hyperthyroidism can include getting lumps in the thyroid (called adenomas) which again can affect the output of the thyroid hormones, inflammation of the thyroid and hormonal imbalances, but again, the most common cause is Grave's disease as mentioned above.

Symptoms
Symptoms can include anxiety, stress, weight loss,

diarrhoea, fast heartbeat, nervousness, increased appetite, tiring easily from using energy quickly, shakes, irritation, menstrual abnormalities, eyes that look as if they are bulging, swollen thyroid (known as 'goitre'), sweating, clammy skin and general weakness.

As you can see these are all things that relate to everything being sped up in the system.

Solutions

Firstly, if it is down to Grave's disease and we know this is classed as an auto immune disease, we should start by looking at the gut because as we have mentioned many times with regards to autoimmune diseases, they tend to start in this area.

So in order to heal and strengthen the gut, see our 'Leaky Gut' section.

Once we are addressing that, or if it is not down to Grave's disease, we should look at stressors on the body.

If the body is in a chronic or severe state of stress (whether that be chemical, emotional or physical) the hormones in the body will be altered, and that can include the thyroid hormones too. For this reason we should ensure that we do what we can to reduce any of these stressors.

- Physical stress - which can come from injuries, pains, burns and other such things

- Emotional stress - which can come from being stressed out, having negative thoughts and being around negative people, worry and anxiety

- Chemical stress - which can come from medications, vaccines, poor diet, pollution and artificial chemicals (in foods, drinks, water supplies, pesticides and things of that nature)

By reducing these or ideally eliminating them completely, we can help our body move out of the sympathetic nervous system state, or 'fight or flight' state, and help it move into the parasympathetic nervous system state, or 'rest and digest' state, which will then not only help in healing the gut as the blood flow and energy can return to this area properly, but will also help the body to balance itself out and repair any damage it may have which will then allow hormones to balance themselves out too.

This should all be accompanied by a diet that is high in fruits, vegetables, nuts, seeds and good fats. You will see this mentioned in the 'Leaky Gut' section also so we advise that you read through that section of the book.

Hypothyroid

What is it?
The opposite of 'hyper'thyroid is 'hypo'thyroid, which means that the metabolism of the processes of the body are much slower than normal.

This form of thyroid problem is much more common than hyperthyroidism.

So, what causes it?
One of the major things that can lead to a hypothyroid condition is an iodine deficiency in the body. Iodine is an essential trace element that is used to help balance the metabolism of your body by working with the thyroid gland (and a range of other tissues and organs). When this is deficient, a lot of serious problems can occur.

Iodine deficiency can be caused by lack of iodine in the diet or from supplementation and can also be caused by a high level of oestrogen in the body and that is because oestrogen actually inhibits the absorption of iodine, which is why we see women affected with this much more than men.

Iodine deficiency can also be caused by having an accumulation of chemicals in the system, especially other 'halogen' elements. Halogens are a group of elements found on the periodic table that includes iodine, chlorine, bromine, astatine, and fluorine.

When any of these elements are present in the body, they interfere with and take the place of iodine and thus lead to an iodine deficiency.

Fluorine, which we come into contact with as Fluoride, is also a neurotoxin and is found in toothpastes, mouthwashes, some water supplies especially in the US, supplements, gels and foams, varnishes and other consumer products and should be avoided at all costs. You can find more information on neurotoxins in our 'Holistic Nervous System Building' section at the beginning of the book.

Chlorine is needed by the body in the form of chloride, but not in high amounts. Having it in high amounts will decrease the efficiency of the iodine. It can be mainly found added in water supplies around the world and as sodium chloride (which is salt, we will talk a little more about salt in the solutions below).

Bromine, encountered by us as bromides, can be found in pesticides, soft drinks, chemicals used for carpets, mattresses and other fabrics, medications and even some bakery foods such as bread dough.

Astatine is generally not one you have to worry about.

Other causes that can lead to a low thyroid hormone production in the system is problems with the kidneys, liver and/or gallbladder as this is where T4 is converted in to T3 (the active version the body needs).

Chronic stress can be a cause of hypothyroidism too because when the body is stressed, whether chemically, emotionally or physically, the body goes into a stressed state known as the sympathetic nervous system, the 'fight or flight' state, which activates stress hormones such as cortisol which if present in high levels in the body, will reduce the amount of T3 (the active thyroid hormone) present.

Finally and another important cause of this condition is a selenium deficiency as this is an essential element for the conversion of T4 into the active form of T3.

Symptoms

Symptoms can include depression, lethargy, constipation, weight gain, fatigue, dry skin, feeling cold a lot, hair thinning and lack of sweating. In extreme cases mental retardation and lack of physical growth.

As you can see these are all related to the slowing down of the processes of the body.

Solutions

There are a whole host of things that can be done to help naturally rebalance an under active thyroid, these would be things like:

- Drinking lots of fresh and filtered water instead of tap water and pre bottled drinks (as these contain other chemicals in them), you can also drink freshly squeezed organic fruit juices and blends too

- Avoid fluoride at all costs. The body just doesn't need it and it has proven through many studies to be a neurotoxin. So why would you risk it? The fact that it is still in toothpastes, mouthwashes, other consumer products and added to millions of people's water supply is just ridiculous and an absolute health hazard

- Don't eat foods with added salt, this would be things like processed and junk foods/drinks. These types of foods and drinks should also not be consumed for the whole host of other chemicals and irritants to the body that they contain

  It is best to avoid normal table salt all together and eat sea salt instead. While table salt and sea salt are both sodium chloride, table salt is highly refined to just contain literally the sodium chloride with 'anti-caking agents', which are further chemicals added so that the salt particles do not stick together

  Sea salt actually retains the trace elements such as zinc, iron and phosphorus amongst others and so doesn't have these sticking problems

  Still be aware of where the sea salt comes from though as it is created by just evaporating sea water. If there is a lot of pollution in the sea waters where it was harvested, there could be concentrations of heavy metals and chemicals in there too, so be aware of that

- A very important one is to eat foods high in iodine such as seaweed (you can get high iodine natural foods in supplement form too)

but again, be careful where you get these from for the reasons mentioned above.

- Always soak your fruit and veg in water and vinegar for 30 minutes before eating them (9 parts water to 1 part vinegar) which will help to dissolve some of the pesticide residues that are left on there

- As we mentioned above, when oestrogen is in too high of a level in the body, the amount of iodine will be decreased. Soy will raise oestrogen levels in the body and as such will decrease iodine levels. So avoid soy and foods containing soy

- Use natural cleaning products and deodorants for both your body and your home

- Ensure to have a sufficient amounts of the trace element selenium which can be obtained from supplements but also naturally from foods such as brazil nuts, mushrooms (button and shiitake), chia seeds, lima beans, seeds (flax, sunflower and sesame) and brown rice

- Avoid large amounts of cruciferous vegetables known as 'goitrogens' as these can further decrease the enzyme called 'thyroid peroxidase' that allows iodine to be used by the thyroid. Cruciferous vegetables are things like broccoli, cauliflower, brussel sprouts and kale

These are packed full of vitamins and minerals though so you can still consume them but not often while having an under active thyroid

- Avoid medications where possible as these are chemicals (if you are on some and want to come off, do so with the supervision of a healthcare professional)

- Exercise regularly to release any accumulated toxins

- Consume unrefined, pure coconut oil as this will help in building cell membranes and boosting enzyme production

- Consume organic foods and drinks that will help to strengthen the liver and kidneys such as beetroot, berries and foods high in Vitamin C and E

- Eat organic, fresh and predominantly raw fruits and vegetables to help detox the body of chemicals and revitalise it with the minerals, enzymes and nutrients it needs to do its job of keeping you strong, healthy and vibrant (this includes nuts, seeds and good fats too)

- Finally, get out in the sun to help keep Vitamin D levels high

Implementing these things will definitely help you on the track back to a balanced and healthy life style where dis-ease is not a concern for you.

Kidney Disease

What is it?
Kidney disease is a chronic condition characterised by the degeneration of the kidneys (the body's natural filtering system for waste products and toxins and it also removes the excess water from the blood).

When the 'nephrons', which are the mini filters in the kidneys, become damaged their ability to filter is compromised and they continue to deteriorate. Waste and chemicals can then accumulate in the blood and kidneys and cause a range of other problems for the body.

So, what causes it?
Some of the causes for kidney disease can be things such as high blood sugar which can damage the capillaries in the kidneys causing them to malfunction. Another big cause is chronic high blood pressure as this weakens, narrows, hardens and puts strain on the arteries around the kidneys which then reduces the oxygen and blood flow to the area.

Other causes can be continuous dehydration as not keeping yourself hydrated can lead to kidney stones and thus blockages leading to malfunctioning kidneys.

Finally, chemicals and toxins in the body can put pressure on the kidneys as they must be filtered through here. This can come from medications, chemicals in processed and junk foods and drinks, heavy metal exposure in water and other such chemical exposures.

Symptoms

Symptoms of kidney disease can include nausea, change in urine production, dark urine, fatigue and weakness, lack of appetite, thirst and dry mouth, muscle soreness, cramps, shortness of breath, sore feet and ankles, confusion and loss in mental sharpness.

Solutions

Things to consider when looking to heal and recover from kidney disease, while a long process, will include things like:

- Reducing all toxins and chemicals coming into the body to help give the kidneys a chance to work without the continuous strain

- Reduce intake of sugar and sugary foods (and foods that turn into sugar such as wheat, grains and other starchy foods)

- Reduce all stresses on the body in all forms, which is chemical (toxins, medications, vaccines, synthetic chemicals), emotional (everyday stresses, negative thoughts, being around negative people and environments) and physical (pains, injuries, damage and other such things) to help the system return to its parasympathetic state which is known as the 'rest and digest' state. In this state, the body can heal much better

- Reduce acidity and dehydrating substances you bring into the system by reducing the acidic foods that you consume (processed and junk foods/drinks and high consumption of animal proteins) and eat lots of alkalising foods to help the body stay in its naturally slightly alkaline state. The less tax you put on the body, the easier it is going to be for the body to rebuild and repair itself

- Drinks lots of fresh and filtered water

- Boost your immune system which you can do by following our 'Holistic Immune System Building' section

- Eat lots of fresh, organic and raw fruits, vegetables, nuts and seeds to get the minerals, vitamins and nutrients into the body that is needed for healthy, well-functioning cells. These will also at the same time help to detox the body of the toxins that may have accumulated

Kidney Stones

What is it?
Kidney stones is a build-up of crystals in the kidneys as the kidneys are used to filter waste as we mentioned in 'Kidney Disease'. The most common type of crystal that forms is the 'calcium oxalate' crystal.

These crystals can then get big enough to become stuck in the kidney or ureter (which is the tube that leads from the kidneys to the bladder).

Men are much more affected by this than women.

So, what causes it?
Kidney stones are caused by things such as dehydration from a high salt diet and lack of water intake, excessive amounts of animal protein which can increase uric acid build up which in turn reduces citrate which helps to reduce the build-up of the most common type of kidney stones, the calcium oxalate (uric acid is also another type of kidney stone that can form).

So low citrate levels, dehydration and a low, acidic pH can lead to kidney stones.

Lots of toxins in the body can also lead to kidney stones by putting excessive tax on the kidneys and dehydrating the body of water and electrolytes. This can be from a poor diet with lots of processed and junk foods/drinks and from other means such as medications, pesticides and other synthetic chemicals in foods/drinks and water.

Other causes can include too much calcium in the kidneys, which can actually be a result of Vitamin D deficiency and/or a less than sufficient parathyroid hormone functioning. UTI's can also lead to this by again blocking the ureters and blocking up the kidney release.

Symptoms

Symptoms can include bad pain in the back where the kidneys are located, pain, burning and possible blood when urinating, feeling sick and throwing up.

Solutions

There are a range of natural foods and drinks that you can consume and things you can do to help dissolve and pass the stones, rehydrate your body and resolve the problem (unless you have very large stones, then you may need further medical help).

Solutions include:

- Celery juice and the seeds also

- Citrus fruits which will help to build up the amount of citrate in the kidneys again

- Drink lots of fresh and filtered water

- Lots of fresh and organic lemons squeezed in water and eating lemons too

- Drink freshly juiced beetroot juice

- Good amounts of fibre in your diet and ensure your diet is not too high in protein

- Reduce salt intake

- Reduce toxins by limiting the amount of toxins you introduce into your body through foods, drinks, water, medications and other synthetic chemicals

- Get sufficient exercise to further help release toxins out of the body

Leaky Gut

What is it?
This is quite a major section of the book and if you have been reading the book all the way through, you will notice that we have recommended on multiple occasions that you come to this section to understand it fully and how it relates to health.

Leaky gut syndrome, which is also known as gastro-intestinal permeability, is a condition whereby the lining of the gut (the small intestines), which has millions of tiny little hairs protruding from it called 'villi' which absorb nutrients from the food you eat, becomes in a sense loose. When this happens, any undigested proteins present in the gut can then pass through this barrier and gain direct access to the blood stream which can cause a wide range of problems as we shall explore below.

So, what causes it?
Leaky gut can be caused by inflammation to the gut, the deterioration of good bacteria there and general poor diet and lifestyle which puts increased pressure on the gut.

Fatty, chemically filled, highly sugary and other acidic foods (such as processed and junk foods) can cause the gut to become inflamed, damage the villi and cause the gut lining to become loose and 'leaky'. These things can also increase the growth of Candida too.

Medications such as antibiotics and the things

mentioned above can destroy the guts ecosystem of good bacteria that helps you break down food and keep your gut in a healthy, working order and can compromise the effectiveness of the immune system as 80% is located in this area too.

Undigested proteins and such are not supposed to enter directly into the bloodstream, only the nutrients from the digested food is supposed to get through by being absorbed by the hair like villi.

- Proteins are supposed to be broken into Amino Acids

- Fats are supposed to be broken down into Fatty Acids and

- Carbohydrates are broken down into Glucose

Vitamins and minerals also become absorbable after being broken down in the intestines.

What this can lead to:
When this happens, the cells can then receive all the nutrients they need in the proper way. When this doesn't happen and the food particles (containing undigested proteins) get through into the blood stream, major problems can occur.

One of the major things that can happen is that the brain can actually be affected in a negative way when the gut is damaged, altered or destroyed. For more on this visit our 'Holistic Nervous System Building' section where you will find the 'Gut-Brain Connection' section.

Many allergies can develop from having a leaky gut and what is known as 'auto-immune diseases' can also develop from this condition.

How?

When these whole undigested proteins slip through into the blood stream they are seen as foreign invaders by the immune cells and an attack is mounted against them.

Antibodies are produced and then when the body see's these proteins again, it will attack it much quicker in an attempt to eliminate it.

The interesting thing is that something called 'molecular mimicry' can also come into play.

Molecular mimicry is essentially the process where the body, after creating antibodies to attack the invader, then believes that it recognises the same invaders in the body somewhere else.

This is because, as we talked about in the 'Body Essentials' section, the body contains thousands of different combinations of proteins doing a wide range of important jobs. Because there are so many different combinations of proteins, if a foreign protein does get in and an attack is mounted against it, there is a high chance that the foreign protein looks like a protein that is already part of the body. As antibodies have been created to fight these off, they will then just attack our proteins that look like the invader too.

This can take place in a range of places, and

depending where that happens this will determine the auto-immune disease and allergy that occurs.

For example, Rheumatoid Arthritis is the immune cells attacking the joints, Grave's Disease is where it attacks the thyroid gland, in Lupus the immune cells can attack any organ of the body, Fibromyalgia is where the immune cells attack the muscles and the list goes on.

It is also interesting to note that literally all Autistic children are known to have chronic problems with their gut too. As you may recall from the 'Holistic Nervous System Building' section near the start, there is a 'gut-brain' connection.

Once we know this is the cause of auto immune disease, and we know the cause of leaky gut, we have much more power to take these conditions into our own hands to find solutions and help for them.

Be sure to also understand 'Candida' and how this can also affect the gut and lead to a leaky gut. Visit our 'Candida' section for more on that.

Symptoms
Symptoms of leaky gut syndrome can include bloating, diarrhoea, constipation, gas, headaches, brain fog and memory loss, excessive fatigue, development of nutritional deficiencies, increasing amounts of newly developing allergies, new development of autoimmune diseases especially with no genetic predisposition and more.

Solutions

Here is an in-depth way to help heal your leaky gut. You can heal your gut bit by bit if you like, but the following recommendation is for those who want to fully and effectively heal, re-close and strengthen the gut and repopulate it with good, healthy bacteria.

Follow this for around 40 days initially whilst keeping an eye on blood pressure too. Evaluate how you feel and then continue if you feel the need too.

As this is a kind of detox as well you may notice symptoms such as headaches, skin break outs, irritability, some bloating and diarrhoea, food cravings, fatigue and some trouble sleeping because your system is flushing out all of the toxins that may have been present.

For this reason, it is important to keep track of your blood pressure and other things such as blood sugar too. If you like, you can do this with the assistant of a healthcare professional (especially if you are on medication).

So let's get into this, we will just list everything below:

We will start with the no's:

No meat & fish, no dairy, no breads, no grains, no added or refined sugars (such as high fructose corn syrup and corn starch), no caffeine, no processed foods, no junk foods, no trans-fats and hydrogenated oils, nothing cooked over 118 degrees (you can lightly steam if you like), no alcohol, no smoking, no artificial sweeteners/colours or preservatives, no fizzy drinks and try and cut out some of the nightshades too as these can cause problems and can delay the healing process of the gut (potatoes, egg-plant, tomatoes, tobacco, peppers)

What's left, right?

Essentially you want to be just eating raw, organic and as fresh as you can fruits and vegetables with some nuts, seeds and good fats.

Trying to eat these as raw as possible will give you the most amount of enzymes, nutrients and healing power. If you can't do them all raw or can't blend/juice them and drink them, then only lightly steam them (but this will still take some of the enzymes out).

We will also include pre and probiotics in there too. But I will list them below.

So the best foods for this cleansing and rebuilding period are these:

Celery, Beetroot, Ginger, Garlic, Parsley (and its root), Kale, Cucumber, Dandelion (its root and greens), Lemon, Cloves, Black Walnut Hulls, Coconut Oil, Papaya (and its seeds), Green Onions, Pineapple, Pumpkin Seeds, Avocado, Krill Oil and/or Algae Oils, Hemp Seeds, Seaweed like Wakame, Chia Seeds and Flax Seeds, Fennel Seed, Cinnamon, Gentian, Liquorice Root, Olives, Oregano, Thyme and Turmeric.

Make sure all of these foods are GMO free, as fresh as possible and organic where possible too. Remember to soak them in water and vinegar (9 parts water to 1 part vinegar) to try and dissolve any of the pesticide residue left on them where appropriate.

You can also eat and/or blend other fruits and vegetables too at this time in abundance, especially dark leafy greens.

You can mix and match these in salads, juices, blends or have them on their own. You can try and get creative with them too to keep it fun and different so you don't get bored of them.

Then along with the foods above it will be beneficial to take the natural pre and probiotics which will help to repopulate your gut with good bacteria and help with healing the gut and getting rid of bad bacteria. These are:

Prebiotics (which help to essentially feed the probiotics and allow them to grow quicker): Fresh Dandelion Greens and Root, Onions, Asparagus, Chicory, Garlic, Burdock, Jerusalem Artichoke, Brussel Sprouts, Cabbage, Cauliflower, Collard Greens, Kale and Radish.

Probiotics are the good bacteria's we want, which are included in: Fermented Vegetables (which includes foods like sauerkraut), Kombucha, Kimchi, Coconut Kefir, Miso and others. You can also get probiotics in supplemental form, but if you go for this option try and find ones without lots of fillers and other chemical additives in with them.

In addition to your diet, another important thing which we have said time and time again throughout this book, will be to reduce the amount of toxins you are exposed to and allow into your body through medications (especially antibiotics), aerosols (can get natural deodorants), toothpastes and mouthwashes (go for a fluoride free one, fluoride can also be in the form of sodium-fluorosilicate as well), washing products for your skin, creams and hair products.

You also want to ensure you are drinking lots of fresh and filtered water too.

Finally, we want to reduce any kinds of stressors on the body, such as chemical, emotional and physical stresses.

- Chemical stresses can include medications, vaccines, toxins, synthetic chemicals, pollution, processed and junk foods

- Emotional stresses can include day to day stress, anxiety, worry, depression and other such emotional disturbances

- Physical stresses can include injuries, pains, strains, traumas and other damage to the system

So to help de-stress, do things like walking and doing exercise which as a bonus will get out more toxins. Meditation is a great tool to de-stress, re-centre and quieten down the mind, yoga is the same and finding and doing other things that relax you will be beneficial as this will speed up the healing.

Other good things to consider is chanting and loud humming. This is because the gut is closely linked to the brain by a nerve called the 'Vagus Nerve'. By stimulating this whilst healing your gut, your brain will also receive the benefits of this type of healing.

The stronger this connection, the better in sync and healthier the nervous system will be and thus the brain and gut too.

By doing this you can move the body into a parasympathetic nervous system state, which is the 'rest and digest' state, rather than continuously being in a sympathetic nervous system state, which is the 'fight or flight' state which essentially is a continuously stressed state that gears the body up for some kind of physical action and takes blood flow and energy away from the digestive system.

Remember to keep checking your progress intermittently and adjusting where needed. Following this plan should definitely help you to heal the gut and thus a wide range of other reactions in the body that stem from this.

Migraine

What is it?
A migraine is a type of neurological disorder in which the nerves become hypersensitive which begins in the 'Trigeminal Nerve' (the nerve that branches off through the face), which is why the symptoms are what they are which are mentioned in the symptoms section.

The chemicals that are produced from the stress on the nerve then releases further chemicals which cause pain and inflammation.

So, what causes it?
As this is related to the nerves, we again have to look at neurotoxins. Neurotoxins are chemicals that affect the nerves predominantly by stimulating and exciting them too much, sometimes to the point of death. This quick firing and hyper excitability can lead to inflammation of the nerves too.

Some neurotoxins to be aware of are things like:

- Fluoride (which is found in many toothpastes, mouthwashes and water supplies)
- Pesticides (sprayed on crops)
- Herbicides and Fungicides (sprayed on crops)
- MSG (Monosodium Glutamate - found in a wide range of foods - as a note, anything that says 'Flavouring' could very much be MSG)
- Aspartame and Sucralose (which are artificial sweeteners found in many foods and drinks - read ALL of your food labels - especially those

things that say 'diet' and 'sugar free')
- Aluminium (found in vaccines, drinking water and medications)
- Mercury (which can be found in water, fish products, vaccines and tooth fillings).

The excessive stimulation of nerves in the head can lead to continued migraine attacks. This can come about from the neurotoxins we mentioned above but also by keeping the body in a continued state of stress, whether that be chemical, emotional or physical.

Other causes for migraine attacks can be lack of sleep or relaxation which causes the body to not produce the right amount of chemicals needed to keep pain at bay.

Finally, genetics can play a role in making some one more prone to the condition, although this does not guarantee that someone will suffer from it.

Symptoms
Symptoms can include throbbing in the head area, sinus pressure, head tenderness, congestion of the sinuses, sore muscles, headaches, light sensitivity, sound sensitivity, nausea, dental pain, neck pain, a blank spot in sight and can have tingling and slight numbness.

Solutions
Firstly, it will be important to get the body out of a stressed state whenever not having a migraine attack,

by doing this the body will have a better chance of healing and detoxing itself and bringing in the nutrients needed for a healthy nervous system.

Next, it will be important to cleanse any accumulation of heavy metals, neurotoxins and other toxic and synthetic chemicals out of the body to allow the nervous system to do its job efficiently without being disrupted by the build-up of chemicals.

You can then strengthen the nervous system too. To see full detailed information on the stressed state, neurotoxins and detoxing of the nervous system, read the 'Holistic Nervous System Building' section of this book.

Multiple Sclerosis (MS)

What is it?

MS is considered as an auto-immune disease in which the body is attacking itself. In MS the immune system starts to attack the 'myelin' that surrounds and protects the nerves of the nervous system. When this continues, it then leads to lesions (scarring). When there is no myelin around the nerve, the signal passing down the nerve is greatly reduced.

So, what causes it?

As this is classed as an auto-immune disease, we must address the gut again. See the 'Leaky Gut' section for full details on how auto-immune diseases are linked to the gut.

As with any problems with the nervous system we must always take into consideration the role neurotoxins play here.

Neurotoxins are chemicals that interfere with the functioning of the nervous system. They excite the neurones sometimes to the point of death and cause inflammation too. For more information on neurotoxins, heavy metals and nervous system health in general read the 'Holistic Nervous System Building' section.

Some to be aware of are Fluoride, Artificial Sweeteners like Aspartame and Sucralose, heavy metals like Mercury and Aluminium and food additives like MSG.

As well as neurotoxins, other toxins that affect the functioning of the body and nervous system are medications, chemicals in processed and junk foods/drinks, chemicals in water supplies and synthetic products used for your body and home.

Symptoms

Symptoms can include fatigue, slurred speech, losing balance, tingling and numbness across the body and spine too, weakness, dizziness, vision problems, depression, poor concentration, memory loss and coordination issues.

Solutions

You can get relief and help heal MS by doing things such as firstly being aware that the cause could very well be from the gut as it is an auto-immune disease, so read the 'Leaky Gut' section on how to go about healing and rectifying that issue.

That section will address diet, so other things will include doing as much exercise as is possible without overdoing what you can manage as this will help you to maintain the system by keeping the lymphatic system moving, blood flowing and oxygen circulating.

You want to also get plenty of deep rest to help the body come out of any kind of stressed state as being in a stressed state (and you can probably say this without reading it now) will keep the body in a sympathetic nervous system state, otherwise known as the 'fight or flight' response and instead we want to help the body get back into the parasympathetic nervous system state, otherwise known as the 'rest and digest' state.

Being in a sympathetic nervous system state is going to take blood supply away from the gut and processes for healing, and put the system in a place where stress hormone levels are raised leading to blood sugar and blood pressure being raised in preparation for you to 'fight' or 'flight'. Blood will also be redirected to the extremities for the same reason and the nervous system will also be heightened in awareness.

- Meditation is one of the best ways in which to get the body out of a stressed state, calm the mind and nervous system, help the body to heal and re-align energies

- Totally eliminate the intake or exposure to toxic chemicals (including medications), neurotoxins and heavy metal as much as you possibly can to stop any further damage being done to the nervous system and immune system

- Eliminate processed and junk food/drink intake which have lots of chemicals, sugar and other things that are not very good for the body and can again put the body into a stressed state and damage the gut further.

- Help cleanse the blood by eating predominantly raw, organic and fresh foods such as garlic, onions, dandelion root, apples, beetroot, parsley, carrots, turmeric root, berries, coriander and a range of dark leafy greens.

- When you eat or juice/blend these foods, remember to eat fruit and vegetables after soaking them in water and vinegar (9 parts water and 1 part vinegar) to remove any pesticide residues.

- Consume good amounts of good fats like krill oil, avocados, olives, nuts, seeds like ground chia and flax and an abundance of coconut oil which helps with the rebuilding of the myelin

- Ensure to have sufficient amount of Vitamin D in your system

Selenium and Vitamin E. As you may have read in our 'Holistic Nervous System Building' section of this book, Selenium is extremely important in creating the enzyme 'Glutathione Peroxidase' which is one of the most important antioxidants and free radical disposers in the body and is paramount to good nerve health.

In MS, a lot of oxidative stress occurs in the neurones and for this reason Selenium should be used. If it is used with the addition of Vitamin E, which acts as another antioxidant in the body, the effect is enhanced and oxidation and free radical damage is reduced.

- Cut out cheap (as it is factory farmed and factory farmed animals generally have lots of antibiotics in them and eat GMO feed), fatty and processed meats. If you eat meat, eat lean and organic, grass fed animals. This also applies to their milk.

Obesity

What is it?

Obesity is the condition of having a lot of excess and unneeded body fat that is very damaging to the system, its organs and its processes.

So, what causes it?

Obesity is not just about eating too much. While that does factor into it, that would not be fair to call that the full picture.

There are a few possible causes but essentially it seems to come down to this chain of events. We will explain all of these in a little more detail.

- Insulin levels become raised in the body initially. They then stay at a relatively raised level
- The cells then lose their receptivity to the insulin
- Insulin can then not open up cells the way it should in order to get energy in (as insulin is like the key that opens up the cell to allow glucose in to be used as energy)
- This increases the overall insulin levels travelling around in the blood and increases the amount of fat stored
- High levels of insulin blocks a chemical called 'Leptin' from reaching the brain

This sequence of events is essentially the major cause and pathway that the majority of people with obesity fall into. Let's look at it a little deeper.

- **Insulin levels become raised in the body initially. They then stay at a relatively raised level**

Insulin is released whenever blood glucose rises. This happens whenever we eat carbohydrates, protein (albeit raising the blood glucose slower) and, of course, things with sugar in. So knowing this, we can clearly see that by having a high starchy carb, high sugar diet, we will increase the amounts of insulin circulating in our blood.

Foods that fall into this category of increasing insulin production are things like:
- high fructose corn syrup, refined and added sugar, syrups and sweeteners (which are all in most processed and junk foods and drinks), sweets and chocolate, concentrated fruit juices, cereals, wheat and anything made with wheat, white potatoes, all fast foods and most processed foods, white rice, fizzy and sweetened drinks, milk, some bottled dressings and other such things. Always check the labels to see.

Just so you are aware, 1 teaspoon is equal to about 4 grams of sugar.

- **The cells then lose their receptivity to insulin**

The reason this happens is because with a constant high level of insulin floating around in the blood, the cells lose their sensitivity to it as its always there, and so over overtime they become 'resistant' to it.

Or in other words, the cells just stop taking up the insulin and thus the glucose the way they should.

- **Insulin can then not open up cells the way it should in order to get energy in**

Insulin acts like a key that opens up the cells and allows the glucose in to be converted into energy. Without the cells accepting this properly, it is hard to get the sufficient amount of energy in for proper functioning and communication to happen between the cells.

- **This increases the overall insulin levels travelling around in the blood and increases the amount of fat stored**

High levels of insulin travelling around in the blood because of high levels of glucose will promote fat storage. This happens because insulin tries to clear up the excessive amounts of glucose in the blood stream by pushing it into fat cells for later use.

- **High levels of insulin blocks a chemical called 'Leptin' from reaching the brain**

This high level of insulin in the blood also causes a chemical produced in fat cells called 'leptin' to be blocked from reaching the brain. This is known as 'leptin resistance'. Leptin acts like a feedback loop between the fat cells around the body and the brain to let the brain know when you have enough fat stores.

When the brain senses low levels of leptin, the brain generates chemicals and signals to make you hungry to bring in more energy and slows down your thyroid hormone production, which slows down your metabolic process to help you store more energy.

Then because this leptin signal is blocked from reaching the brain, the brain always things you have low levels of leptin and so continues to produce those chemicals and signals.

If the same type of food is entering the body, the cycle will continue.

This is why people who are obese may be always hungry, gain weight quickly and find it hard to stop. The brain cannot see what is really happening in the body to efficiently dictate what needs to happen.

Another cause that revolves around the same type of process is fructose. Now while fructose may come from fruits, we are really talking about the high fructose corn syrup and other concentrated amounts of it found in processed and junk foods and added sugars the world over.

Fructose goes straight to the liver which can alter the pathways of communication in the liver. This condition is known as 'fatty liver'. This too can cause insulin resistance and this forces the pancreas to create more insulin to try and get the liver to accept and take in energy where it is needed.

Obesity is not generally a case of just pure gluttony or anything else, but a cascade of events that can quickly get out of hand.

You will also notice that in the list of foods we gave in

number 1 that we did not mention vegetables, fruits, nuts, seeds and good fats. You will see then that processed and junk foods are not needed by the body, but the vegetables, fruit, nuts, seeds and good fats provide all the nutrients the body needs. These nutrients are used in building healthy cells, strengthening communication channels and keeping the body functioning well.

So the case for obesity... is also one of malnutrition.

Again, this may sound paradoxical, but by eating all of the wrong foods, you are not getting what you need and so the body comes into all sorts of problems.

Other things that play a role and affect leptin and insulin signalling are living a sedentary lifestyle (not much physical activity), stress and overeating of these wrong foods.

Solutions
First and foremost, we want to address the general initial cause of the cascading events that is obesity.

The first is the types of foods that we consume.

- Cut out all processed, junk and foods that are deficient in vitamins and minerals that the body needs.

- Take out the bad fats such as fatty and cheap meats (if you are going to eat meat, eat organic, lean and grass fed meats and wild caught fish, but be sure that the fish comes from a sea that is not contaminated), trans-fats and hydrogenated oils which are found in processed foods, junk foods, fried foods and other snacks.

- Cut out sugary foods and foods that turn to sugar. These include added sugar foods, syrups, sweeteners (artificial and natural), wheat and foods made with wheat, white rice, cereal (which is a processed food), white potatoes and other starchy foods.

With these foods limited or eliminated, we can now rebuild the cells and clear the system up with other foods and actions.

We want to eat as much organic, fresh and predominantly raw fruits, vegetables (vegetables more than the fruits, especially dark leafy greens), nuts, seeds, good fats, fresh herbs and spices as we can.

When we say good fats, these are things like coconut oil (to get your saturated fat which the body needs), olives, avocados, nuts and seeds.

We also want to ensure we have sufficient amounts of omega 3 fatty acids in the system too. These can be obtained from fish and fish oils, algae oil, flax seeds, chia seeds, hemp seeds and seaweed such as wakame.

The best fruits with the lowest impact on your sugar levels, and thus insulin levels, will be things like lemons, limes, berries and watermelon and this is the whole fruit, not concentrated or pre bottled juices.

Include lots of fresh and filtered water and also lots of Vitamin C and D. The best source of vitamin D is of course the sun, but in areas where this is not always possible you can get it in supplemental form using vitamin D3.

Vitamin C can be obtained from, and this is kind of perfect for this solution, dark leafy greens, peppers (bell, chilli), kale, broccoli, cauliflower and berries. All of these will also keep your sugar load down while substantially increasing your vitamin and mineral value.

If you are on cholesterol lowering medications (statins), you want to do your best to come off of these. This solution will definitely help you to lower your cholesterol naturally and thus make it easier to come off of the medication. Try and reduce and come off of other medications too in an attempt to speed up the process of reducing weight by moving the body out of a chemically stressed state. Being in a chemically stressed state also alters the functioning of the cells and how they communicate. Remember to do this with the supervision of a healthcare professional.

As we talk about much deeper in the 'High Cholesterol' section, every single cell of the many trillions the body has needs cholesterol to function correctly and for the production of Vitamin D and your natural steroidal hormones. Lowering it artificially is not a good thing to do and will cause a range of other problems in the system.

We want to make sure that you are absorbing all of

these good nutrients suggested above into your body, for this reason be sure to check out our 'Leaky Gut' page to learn about the importance of the gut in most aspects of health.

Finally, reduce your intake of dairy as this actually promotes the production of mucus and milk actually contains a lot of sugar too. Not to mention if it is not from an organic, grass fed source it will contain GMO proteins too.

Parkinson's Disease

What is it?
Parkinson's disease is a progressive neurological disease that breaks down the neurones that transmit dopamine in the brain. Dopamine levels then drop and the smooth movement of muscles does not happen the way it should.

As it is a progressive condition, it means it gradually gets worse over time.

So, what causes it?
The causes of Parkinson's, and a few of the other conditions mentioned in this book, have been said to have no known cause or cure in current mainstream healthcare.

But let's look at Parkinson's. We know that the amount of neurotoxins, chemicals, GMO foods and other toxins we have been consuming through the environment, foods, water and air have been on the rise especially in the last 10 years. This is also true for Parkinson's disease.

As Parkinson's is a neurological disease, it would make sense to first look at these neurotoxins that are in our foods, water, air and soils.

We have gone into this in more detail in the 'Holistic Nervous System Building' section of the book, but some neurotoxins to be aware of are things like:

- Fluoride (which is found in many toothpastes,

mouthwashes and water supplies)
- Pesticides (sprayed on food crops)
- Herbicides and Fungicides (sprayed on food crops)
- MSG (Monosodium Glutamate - found in a wide range of foods - as a note, anything that says 'Flavouring' could very much be MSG)
- Aspartame and Sucralose (which are artificial sweeteners found in many foods and drinks - read ALL of your food labels - especially those things that say 'diet' and 'sugar free')
- Aluminium (found in vaccines, drinking water and medications)
- Mercury (which can be found in water, fish products, vaccines and tooth fillings)

Heavy metals and neurotoxins are definitely the first place to look when looking at neurological diseases.

By definition these kinds of chemicals interfere with the neurones and cause hyper excitability which can cause all kinds of problems, worst of all being death of the neurones.

We then should look at any traumas, other than the chemically induced, that the neurones may have sustained. Such as external injuries and problems that may have occurred.

As age increases, you are also more likely to get Parkinson's disease as the nervous system starts to deteriorate.

Symptoms

Symptoms can include tremors and shaking in hands, legs and arms, stiff muscles, balance problems and slower movements.

Solutions

To help with the deterioration of Parkinson's it is advisable to try and look after the nervous system and do what you can to keep it healthy and strong, for full detailed information on that, see our 'Holistic Nervous System Building' section.

Avoid all neurotoxic chemicals (including heavy metals), GMO foods, processed foods, junk foods, inorganic foods where possible, added sugar in foods (and food that turns to sugar) and ensure you have a healthy functioning gut to avoid any nutritional deficiencies. For more on the gut, see our 'Leaky Gut' section.

Be sure to boost your intake of Vitamin D too which is paramount to a healthy nervous system.

Finally, you want to ensure that the body is not unnecessarily in a stressed state, whether that be chemically, emotionally or physically. Keeping the body in a stressed state will cause the deterioration to happen much quicker than otherwise.

Please be sure to have a read of our 'Holistic Nervous System Building' section where you will get full information on how to keep the nervous system functioning well.

Through these methods, it is possible to reduce the

impact of Parkinson's Disease.

Pneumonia

What is it?
Pneumonia is an infection of the alveoli (air pockets in the lungs) that leads to inflammation and then the lungs filling with fluid.

So, what causes it?
It can be caused by a bacterial infection from a bacteria called 'Streptococcus Pneumoniae' and other bacteria's. This is the most common cause.

It can also be caused by the Flu virus, which is actually the main reason why people die from the flu because the immune system is much lower while it fights off the flu or cold and then the bacteria has the opportunity to set in. Finally, fungal infections can cause it too.

Symptoms
Symptoms can include a chesty, heavy, mucus filled cough, fever, fatigue, sore throat, chest pain, muscle aching and shortness of breath.

Solutions
There are a range of things you can do to treat this naturally at the early stages of contraction. This will be things like:

- Cutting out smoking and drinking alcohol

- Avoiding inhalation of other types of smoke, especially indoors

- Keep good hygiene (as the bacteria is passed from person to person)

- Stay away from people who already have the condition

- Ensure to consume high doses of Vitamin C, its ok to consume high amounts because Vitamin C is water soluble and so needs to be replenished often anyway. This will help a lot with pneumonia

- Ensure to have a high levels of Vitamin D, which can be obtained from sun exposure or failing that supplements. This along with the Vitamin C will help to prevent you getting the Flu and Colds by keeping the immune system strong and so keeping bacteria's and viruses at bay

A great method you can add into your daily routine is to get a bowl of steaming hot water with a few drops of tea tree oil in it, put a towel over your head and over the bowl and inhale deeply to fill the lungs with the vapour. Tea tree is very anti-bacterial and can help to clear any mucus and kill off bacteria that is present.

By having proper nutrition to keep the immune system functioning at its best is probably the best way to help you avoid getting pneumonia, and if you have already contracted it, will help in recovering from it. See our 'Holistic Immune System Building' section for full details on how to do that.

This does not mean that if you have a severe case of pneumonia you should not seek medical advice, but if it is in its early stages, you can indeed get rid of it using natural methods.

Polycystic Ovaries Syndrome (PCOS)

What is it?
Polycystic ovaries is a condition whereby the endocrine system is out of balance, specifically the hormones oestrogen and progesterone and an increase in androgen (male hormone).

Eggs that are normally released regularly begin to mature and stay in the ovaries surrounded by some fluid. These then build up without being released and can lead to infertility and other reproductive organ problems.

So, what causes it?
There are three main factors that can lead to PCOS:

- A lack of iodine in the system and raised oestrogen levels can lead to PCOS, which can cause fibroids in women too

- High insulin levels can cause PCOS

- Chronic stress and overactive adrenals can also cause the hormones to become imbalanced and thus cause PCOS

The symptoms listed below come from the hormonal imbalance.

Symptoms

Due to increase in the male sex hormone (androgens) women with polycystic ovaries can experience facial and bodily hair growth, irregular periods (most stop all together while others have light periods or very heavy periods sporadically), acne, pain in abdominal area, weight gain, fertility issues and slightly deeper voice.

Solutions

- Increase intake of iodine through seaweed or supplements and other iodine rich foods

- Reduce sugar intake (and foods that turn to sugar such as white rice, white flour and other wheat products, white potatoes and other starchy foods)

As iodine will be removed from its place by other 'Halogen' elements, it is advisable to avoid:

- Fluoride (found in toothpastes, mouthwashes, water supplies, pesticides and more)

- Chlorine (from tap water and table salt – you can use sea salt instead) and

- Bromide (used as fire retardants in many household items like chairs, carpets, rugs and included in some baked goods too)

Ensure to de-stress in daily life and help to keep the body out of a stressed state (chemically, emotionally and physically) as this will keep the body in an unbalanced state.

- Chemically would be things like toxins, toxic chemicals, neurotoxins, processed and junk foods/drinks, GMO foods and other such harmful substances

- Emotionally would be things like daily stressful situations, anxiety, depression, worries and fear

- Physically would be physical injuries, damage, pain and strains on the body

Eat lots of fresh, organic and predominantly raw fruits and vegetables to help rebalance the hormones and give the body all of the nutrients it needs to stay strong, healthy and vibrant. This should also include nuts, seeds and good fats. To see a full list of the foods included here, view our 'Body Essentials' section near the start of the book.

Get good amounts of daily exercise to help get toxins out of the body through sweat and stimulating the lymphatic system and have a look into meditation as this can be a very powerful way to relax the body and rebalance hormones too.

If you are taking medications, it is always advisable to do what you can to come off of these, but never go 'cold turkey' and just stop. Always do it with the supervision of a healthcare professional.

Psoriasis

What is it?
Psoriasis is a skin condition that displays on the body as rashes and scaly skin. An inflammatory condition where the skin cells reproduce at a very fast rate compared to normal and so build up on the surface on the skin.

So, what causes it?
Generally skin conditions signal to us that there are some type of toxins in the blood and body that the body is trying to throw out through its nearest exit amongst others, which is the skin.

For this reason, we must look at things such as toxicity from chemicals, foods/drinks and other environmental toxins that are getting into the body.

Once this has been addressed or ruled out, we should then look at the GI Tract (intestines etc) to see if toxins and other undigested particles are getting through into the body from here.

It is known that the group of foods known as 'nightshades' can aggravate the intestines and as such cause 'Leaky Gut' which can lead to allergies, negative reactions and auto-immune diseases. Nightshades include things like potatoes, egg-plant, tomatoes, tobacco and peppers.

For more info on how the gut can be linked to these things, see our 'Leaky Gut' section.

Other causes can be stress, infections in the body and intestines and too much sugar which can also aggravate the intestines by increasing the growth of bad bacteria which can damage the gut lining.

Symptoms

Symptoms can include dry, scaly and flaking skin, itchiness, redness and the skin being sore in these areas.

Solutions

There are a range of things you can do to reduce and get rid of psoriasis naturally.

Some are topical (applied to the outside) such as washing the skin with light and natural soaps which will help to stop the build-up of the excess cells and moisturising well after washing with natural oils such as coconut oil and almond oil.

Avoid cold weather where possible, or wrap up well, to help stop the skin drying out.

Then there are internal steps that can be taken such as addressing and fixing a 'Leaky Gut'. Again, for more info on that read our 'Leaky Gut' section. On this page it will give you a range of foods to eat and not to eat and pre and probiotics that will not only help to strengthen the gut quickly, but will also help in getting toxins out of your system and blood at the same time.

Ensure to get good amounts of oxygen to the skin and sunlight. This will help keep a good blood flow to the skin and also help keep your levels of Vitamin D up which is essential for a healthy functioning body.

Reduce stresses on the body. This is in the form of chemicals, emotions and physical stresses.

- Chemical stresses can include medications, toxic chemicals, neurotoxins, environmental toxins, processed and junks foods/drinks and synthetic cleaning products for your body and home

- Emotional stresses can include stresses in day to day life, negative thoughts, being around negative people, worry, anxiety, depression and other such factors

- Physical stresses can include things like injury, damage and pain inflicted on the body (which can be internally and/or externally)

When the body is in any of the stressed states mentioned above, healing, gut repair and digestion are reduced.

Eating healthy, fresh and organic foods wherever possible and drinking lots of fresh and filtered water will help to give the body the vitamins, minerals and nutrients it needs to build healthy, strong cells, organs and defences. This also includes nuts, seeds and good fats.

Cut out all nightshade foods during your healing period to accelerate the rate of healing. Again, these are potatoes, tomatoes, tobacco, egg-plant and peppers.

Avoid fatty, cheap and processed meats and foods. This is because most 'cheap meat' are factory farmed where animals live in close quarters and because of this have lots of antibiotics in their system. They are also fed GMO feed and have growth hormones to fatten them up quicker. This will then all be included in the meat and milk you consume and not be conducive to good health.

So only eat organic and lean meat if possible, although we recommend cutting out meat during this healing period.

Cut out sugar (and things that turn to sugar) but fruits are ok because they come with fibre, vitamins, minerals and antioxidants which do not have the same impact as extracted and refined sugars. It is still best to limit lots of citrus fruits and have more vegetables in your diet, especially dark leafy green vegetables too.

Finally, cut out alcohol, smoking and fried foods as these add more stresses and damage to the body, which is what we are trying to avoid at the moment.

By following these steps you can rapidly see a marked difference in the condition.

Rheumatoid Arthritis (RA)

What is it?
Rheumatoid Arthritis is considered an auto-immune disease which means that the immune cells of the body have started to attack another part of the body in some way.

In the case of RA the immune cells attack the joints and organs. When this happens in the joints, this then leads to inflammation, fluid build-up, swelling and lots of pain.

As the condition worsens, deformity of the fingers and toes can become prevalent.

So, what causes it?
RA, like most other auto immune diseases, stems from the gut in most cases.

The gut develops gaps in it that lets undigested proteins through into the blood stream which should not happen. This then causes the body to mount a defence and attack the protein which later can turn into the body attacking itself as this invading protein can look like other proteins in our system. For more info on just how this works, see our 'Leaky Gut' section.

Genetics can make someone more prone to developing auto-immune diseases, but does not always mean they will actually get it.

Symptoms

Symptoms can include swelling, inflammation, pain, soreness, stiffness, deformity of extremities, fatigue, mirror of joints affected (for example, if left knee is affected, the right knee will be too. If left fingers are affected, right fingers will be too).

Solutions

As this is an auto-immune disease, we must first look at and begin to heal the gut. For more on how to do this, please see our 'Leaky Gut' section.

As the gut is more than likely damaged at this point, it may be easier to juice and/or blend the foods we recommend in the 'Leaky Gut' section to get the nutrients into your system more efficiently.

Do what you can to completely move yourself away from any toxic chemicals, heavy metals, neurotoxins and other environmental toxins which can be found in processed and junk foods/drinks and other such things.

Remember to always soak your fruit and veg in vinegar and water (1 part vinegar to 9 parts water) to help dissolve pesticide residue where possible.

To help further, be sure to include both Vitamin E and Selenium in your detoxing plans.

Get lots of antioxidants into your body such as berries, cherries, celery and cucumber then lots of organic turmeric root and foods like chlorella and spirulina which are packed full of nutrients.

If you have been reading through the whole book, you will see that time and time again we have been saying you must ensure to reduce the amount of stresses on the body and that is because this is very important in helping put the body into an environment that is conducive to healing and good health.

Remember, this is of all stresses: chemical, emotional and physical.

Ensure to have high amounts of Vitamin C and D. It is important to have sufficient amounts of all the vitamins and minerals of course, but when healing Vitamin C and D are essential. So ensure to have high amounts of these in your system at all times.

Although the pain can be extremely bad at times, try your best to keep the body moving. This will help to stimulate the lymphatic system, keep the blood from stagnating and also keep the oxygen flowing to the cells of the body.

Finally, you want to try and come off of your medications, as this is a chemical stressor to the body and adds toxins to the system. Remember, never just stop taking medications and always do this with the supervision of a healthcare professional.

Putting these measures and actions into place will definitely help you in combating your Rheumatoid Arthritis.

Sinus Infections

What is it?

A sinus infection can generally happen when the sinuses first become inflamed and start to swell. This then blocks the drainage areas in the sinus and so fluid starts to build up here. When this happens the fluid that has built up then becomes infected with bacteria.

So, what causes it?

This initial inflammation and swelling can come about from issues such as a deviated septum (which is when the wall that separates the nostrils becomes misaligned in some way).

It can also be caused by excessive mucus build up in the sinus areas from things such as consuming foods that promote and form mucus production.

This will be things such as all dairy products, fatty foods, sugary foods/drinks and foods/drinks with lots of added sugar (and foods that turn to sugar such as wheat, white rice, white potatoes, processed and junks foods), highly acid foods such as meats (especially processed, fatty and/or cheap meats), alcohol, fried foods and caffeine.

Smoking can also impair the lungs abilities to clean itself out, amongst a range of other things that are not healthy for the body.

Also a low immune system can cause you to get cold and flu viruses which then lower the immune system even more and open the way for more bacteria to enter into the sinus which at this time is already filled with mucus, making it a perfect breeding ground for them.

Symptoms

Symptoms can include pain and tenderness in the sinuses and head area, heavy head, congestion, dark mucus, foul smell, pressure in the head, headaches and a tickling throat.

Solutions

First we can try and address the mucus build up and cleanse this out to reduce the infection.

This can be done through things such as a 'Neti Pot'. A neti pot is a plastic pot that is filled with warm salt water and poured into one nostril whilst holding the head forward and letting the liquid drain out of the other side. This is very good for cleansing out excess mucus and, with the addition of the salt, helps to kill any infections that may be present.

Along with the Neti Pot, another good method is to get a steaming bowl of hot water, put a few drops of tea tree oil in it and then get a towel and put it over the head and the bowl. The vapours are then inhaled deeply which will help to clear out excess mucus in the lungs and sinuses. Tea tree oil is very anti-bacterial and so will also help to kill off the bacteria's present in the sinuses.

Eating hot foods like soups will also help to break up

the mucus and as always it is important to drink lots of fresh and filtered water to keep the body hydrated which will stop thick mucus from forming as much.

Avoid the foods that we mentioned above in the causes section. Doing this while taking the measures above will definitely help you to kill the infection and clear your sinuses.

Stroke

What is it?
A stoke is when rapid death occurs in brain tissue due to a disturbance in blood flow to the brain.

This can be in the form of an 'Ischemic' stroke, which is a loss of blood flow to the brain or a 'Hemorrhagic' stroke in which there is bleeding in or on the brain.

Generally in most people's case, stokes are Ischemic.

So, what causes it?
There are many causes for stroke, such as:

- Thrombosis (talked about in the next condition), but essentially this means there is an obstruction of the arteries - whether large or small - due to hardening, thickening or disease of the arterial wall that leads to the brain which then starves the brain of blood and oxygen

- Uncontrolled Hypertension (high blood pressure). This happens because when it is prolonged the constant high pressure can damage the inner lining of the arterial walls.

- 'Hemorrhagic Clots' is another cause that happens elsewhere in the body. This can then break off and travel through the blood stream to that specific artery leading to the brain (this is known as an embolism). This can also happen from congested heart failure and heart attacks

- Septicaemia. An infection in the blood stream and/or heart which can make its way into the arteries and thus up into the brain

Other causes can include a loss of a lot of blood somewhere in the body, traumas to the brain, drug abuse (such as cocaine and methamphetamine), smoking, alcohol abuse, genetic defects, oestrogen deficiency (particularly in menopausal females), medication use and overuse such as anticoagulants (to stop blood from sticking) and other such drugs.

Finally, previous strokes will increase chances of getting another one.

Symptoms

One of the most important symptoms of stroke to look out for is 'F.A.S.T'. Fast stands for:

F = Face. Look to see if their face has drooped on one side.
A = Arms. Can they lift both arms up?
S = Speech. Can they talk and/or is their speech slurred?
T = Time. While not a symptom, the reaction must be quick when someone has a stroke as brain cells are dying every second while this is occurring.

The faster the reaction, the better chance of survival without extensive damage.

Other symptoms can include loss of sensation and movement. Depending on what area of the brain is affected will generally determine the symptoms experienced. It generally takes place on one side of the body and eye sight can go on just one side too. Then they could also have loss of coordination, sudden dizziness and headache.

Solutions

If someone is having a stroke, the only solution is to act fast and get them to a hospital immediately. The longer it goes on the more chance of detrimental damage.

But there are things you can do to prevent the onset of a stroke (which is similar to the solution for heart disease), such as:

-   Ensure to keep the blood clean and oxygenated

-   Remove toxins from the body and do not add more in, this is in the form of medications, drugs, smoking, alcohol, processed and toxic foods/drinks, chemically filled water and avoid air pollution where possible

-   Try to keep the body out of a continuous stressed state in the form of chemical stress (from the things listed above), emotional stress (from negative thoughts, negative people, stressful environments, anxiety and depression) and physical stress (from injuries, damage to the body and physical pains).

Follow the solution listed in the 'Hypertension' section

also to ensure you do not continuously have high blood pressure because of its damaging effects.

- Lower your salt intake, especially from table salt and products with added salt (have sea salt in lower doses instead)

- Lose any excessive weight to take unnecessary strain off of the body

- Ensure to get plenty of rest as the body heals and repairs during deep sleep

- Reduce caffeine intake as it is acidic and dries out the body

- Eat lots of fresh, organic and raw fruits and vegetables to help give the body the vitamins, minerals and nutrients it needs to keep the body strong and healthy. Juice and blend where possible and include nuts, seeds and good fats too.

Consuming lots of Vitamin D and C is vital to a strong and healthy immune system that can help to clear up problems that occur. These vitamins also work to keep all of the cells of the body healthy and vibrant too.

Finally, Selenium is also an important trace mineral that should be taken to protect the neurones from oxidative damage that can happen in the case of stroke. This can then reduce the amount of damage that is caused by any potential stroke.

Thrombosis

What is it?
Thrombosis is essentially a blood clot that occurs in a vein, artery or the heart. You may have heard of 'deep vein thrombosis' which occurs in a vein, generally in the legs.

The clot can cause full or partial blocking of the blood vessels around the body. When this happens, swelling and pain occurs due to the blockage and pressure build up.

So, what causes it?
There are a wide range of causes for thrombosis, such as slowing of blood flow, lack of exercise and movement, being overweight, smoking, cancer, medications that cause the blood to clot, injury to the area such as a severe bruise, trauma or fracture. Anything else that can cause the blood to stagnate has the potential to make the blood clot unnaturally and then cause thrombosis.

It can be caused by a damaged blood vessel wall, unhealthy, fatty, processed and junk foods/drinks and toxins that can all cause narrowing of the arteries and veins from plaque build-up and thus clots can form.

Symptoms
Some people may not experience symptoms, but others can experience pain in the area, tenderness, swelling in the extremities and other such things.

Solutions

You want to get lots of good exercise to help increase the blood flow and oxygen circulation to ensure the clot does not build up any further.

Reduce intake of toxins into the body such as smoking, alcohol, fatty, junk and processed foods/drinks, fried foods, sugary foods (and foods that turn to sugar like white rice, wheat, white potatoes and other starchy foods), medications where possible as this adds toxins to the bloodstream, tap water as this often contains traces of chemicals and finally other toxic products such as those for cleaning the body or home.

If overweight, try and lose the excess weight to help reduce strain on the body and blood vessels.

Drinks lots of fresh and filtered water and lots of fresh, organic and raw fruits and vegetables, especially dark leafy greens. This includes nuts, seeds and good fats too.

Eat foods and have drinks that help to cleanse the blood such as garlic, squeezed lemon and water, green leafy vegetable juices (such as kale and greens), green tea's, pomegranate seed, beetroot, bitter gourd, avocados, apples, hemp seeds, turmeric root, cucumber, burdock root, celery, parsley and coriander. You can mix and match these in blends and juices or just eat them raw to help with the condition.

Tuberculosis

What is it?
Tuberculosis is a bacterial infection that can be transmitted through airborne means and is more predominant is less developed countries due to poor hygiene and lots of people living closely together.

It generally begins in the lungs but can spread to other organs around the body.

So, what causes it?
This again, as with other bacterial infections, comes down to a weakened immune system. You are also at more risk when near places with stagnant water sources, near people who have already contracted the infection and other such means.

Symptoms
Symptoms can include poor appetite, weight loss, chesty and persistent cough, fever, sweating, chest pain and fatigue.

Solutions
There are a range of things you can do to try and suppress and eradicate the bacterial infection, especially if caught very early, such as taking papaya leaves, which have been found to be quite beneficial in such cases as they are very anti-bacterial and immune boosting. Garlic and onions are also very anti-bacterial and strengthening for the immune

system.

- Ginseng strengthens the lungs and immune system

- Propolis strengthens the thymus (where white blood cells mature) and the rest of the immune system

- Barberry is also very anti-bacterial

Other useful foods include liquorice root, pineapple, horsetail, black pepper, lots of Vitamin D, C, E, alma, astragalus and selenium.

While very specific, these have been found to work well in boosting the immunity and fighting off such bacterial infections.

If caught in the early stages, getting a bowl of steaming hot water, putting a few drops of tea tree oil in the bowl and then putting a towel over the head and the bowl whilst inhaling deeply until the stream stops is very beneficial in fighting bacteria in the lungs and sinuses and breaking down and helping to remove excessive mucus.

To get full detailed information on how to boost the immune system, please visit our 'Holistic Immune System Building' section.

Final Words

So that's it!

Now this book is not the be all and end all of healthcare by any means but I truly believe that if you implement these strategies and do your best to commit yourself to them, you will notice a great difference in your health and wellbeing and together through our personal actions we can reduce the increasing cases of these epidemic diseases we are seeing in our societies today.

For all of the solutions mentioned in this book we must be aware that these are not 'overnight cures' but ideas, concepts and techniques that should be factored in to your daily life and sustained for long periods. For some, you may notice a difference very quickly and for others it may take a little more time.

This is also dependant on the severity of your condition and the length of time you have had it for. The earlier you start acting to alleviate any condition you may have, the better and quicker the recovery.

This book should just act as a starting place and I genuinely hope it sparks your interest to begin to look deeper into nutrition, the workings of the body with regards to health and other such subjects.

Many of the solutions here are essentially the ideal paths to follow, a road map if you like, so don't feel discouraged if you can not fully stick to them straight away. Instead they should be guide posts and seen as something to work towards at which ever pace you feel fit. Gradually making changes in these directions will still help you.

It really is a fascinating subject to understand this internal universe in which we have control over and it is the reason I started looking into this in the first place.

It is an ongoing journey of learning that I think will continue for many, many years and I hope, that if you are not on this journey yet, this book may help you begin that journey. If you have already began this journey, I hope this book has further increased your already accumulating knowledge and interest.

Personally, I think that natural therapies should and will rise to the top of mainstream healthcare as people continue to see the benefits and results and continue to think about their long term health and not just short term fixes.

I also personally think that nutrition, energy healing and meditation practices are really the ideal combination of factors for great health, longevity and increasing internal happiness and I would personally recommend exploring and testing out each and coming up with your own conclusions.

Again, thank you for reading this book and I wish you well on your healing journey!

All the best!

www.ingramcontent.com/pod-product-compliance
Lightning Source LLC
Chambersburg PA
CBHW062201270326
41930CB00009B/1606